The
T'ai-Chi Ch'uan
Experience

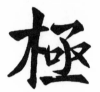

T'ai-Chi Ch'uan
Wu Style

Calligraphy by
Liu Cheng Yü

The T'ai-Chi Ch'uan Experience

Reflections and Perceptions
on Body-Mind Harmony

Collected Essays
Form—Spirit
Philosophy—Structure

Sophia Delza

Foreword by Robert Cummings Neville
Drawings by the Author
Photographs by Lisa Lewicki

STATE UNIVERSITY OF NEW YORK PRESS

Published by
State University of New York Press, Albany

For information, address State University of New York Press,
State University Plaza, Albany, N.Y., 12246

Production by Marilyn P. Semerad
Marketing by Bernadette LaManna

Library of Congress Cataloging-in-Publication Data

Delza, Sophia.
    The T'ai-chi ch'uan experience : reflections and perceptions on
body-mind harmony / Sophia Delza : foreword by Robert C. Neville ;
drawings by the author : photographs by Lisa Lewicki.
        p.   cm.
    Includes index.
    ISBN 0-7914-2897-4 (alk. paper). — ISBN 0-7914-2898-2 (pbk. :
alk. paper)
    1. T'ai chi ch'uan.   I. Title.
GV504.D46   1996
613.7'148—dc20   96-3633
                                                                   CIP

10   9   8   7   6   5   4   3   2   1

This book is dedicated to:

—Grand-master Ma Yueh-Liang, my master-teacher, whose superior wisdom and warm personality laid a secure foundation for me to develop the higher aspects of T'ai-Chi Ch'uan, I offer my respect and devotion.

—The memory of my husband, A. Cook-Glassgold, who made it possible for me to live and study in China . . . never to forget.

—To all of my students, whose integrity and sustained perseverance to attain and comprehend the ultimate harmony of T'ai-Chi Ch'uan elevated and inspired my teaching 'Way.'

Contents

List of Illustrations and Tables

Tables

Foreword

Sophia Delza calls T'ai-Chi Ch'uan an "exercise-art."[1] This is a felicitous if symbolic expression for a Chinese idea that has no elegant English equivalent. Most Westerners who know T'ai-Chi Ch'uan at all call it a martial art, by which they mean a fighting style. But the Chinese martial arts (*wu shu*—see Chapter VII) are much more than fighting styles. They go beyond skill at winning to disciplines aimed at perfecting a person's body and mind, personal relationships, and even community. Victory in a fight can be discerned fairly easily. Excellence of body and mind, and of human relations and community, is more difficult to discern or describe, and its criteria are closer to those of art than they are to those of power. This is part of the reason to call T'ai-Chi Ch'uan an exercise-art.

Actually, to call T'ai-Chi Ch'uan a martial art at all is misleading, as Ms Delza points out in Chapters VII and VIII. Its spirit and techniques are not at all aggressive, and it can be played perfectly by one person alone. Of course, the performance of T'ai-Chi Ch'uan can be entertainment and instruction; a good performance is high art.[2] Its moves sometimes can be used in self-defense, mainly as strategies for getting out of the way. The Taoist philosophy in T'ai-Chi Ch'uan advocates bending, ducking, and running away, rather than fighting to win. T'ai-Chi Ch'uan practice is not for the sake of winning anything but for the sake of its own perfection. It is an exercise for the sake of its own exercise, another part of the reason to call it an exercise-art.

Sophia Delza's essays and poems in this volume arise from her long spiritual as well as physical practice and teaching of T'ai-Chi Ch'uan. She has taken T'ai-Chi Ch'uan to heart and lived with it. As she makes clear here, practicing the physical movements of the exercise-art has effects on one's mental and emotional life, in one's personal relations, and on one's whole style of life. T'ai-Chi Ch'uan is not a religion, but it has great spiritual depths that affect religious as well as political and ethical dimensions of life. These essays, then, reflect far more than her understanding merely of the exercise-art, but rather also her understanding of life. Not least important in that understanding is her refusal to take herself too seriously: there are no black belts for the T'ai-Chi Ch'uan player! The lighthearted poems are as important as the heavy historical essays.

Another reason to call T'ai-Chi Ch'uan an exercise-art relates to the Chinese sensibility regarding the practices or habitual exercises designed to make one's life itself a work of art. Not a work of art in the common Western sense, but in a unique Chinese sense. The Western sense of the word sugests that an object of art is somehow framed, dislocated from its context, isolated, or called attention to in its own terms. Whereas Western *ethical* sensibilities most often connect things in means-ends continua, subordinating one thing to another in orders of justice and in service to human flourishing, Western *aesthetic* sensibilities run against this grain by calling attention to what things are in themselves, what their own qualities are, how the world seems as an environment for them irrespective of their instrumental places in the humanized world. Western aesthetic sensibilities strive to seize the particular and break the tyranny of moral contextualizing. The tension between morals and art in the West is not difficult to discern or even to understand.[3]

A different sensibility regarding both morals and art obtains in East Asia. A work of art is a focal point for harmonizing, and harmonizing with, its environment. A fine painting, a graceful ceramic bowl, or a brilliantly danced piece in Classical

Chinese Theater is aimed to define the space it is in. It does not create a "virtual" environment (to use computer jargon) as a work of art in a Western museum might, but engages its real environment. Or rather, the Chinese sensibility about art looks to how a work engages its real environment, whereas the Western sensibility looks to how a work of art creates a virtual environment for itself in tension with its actual moral implications. The Chinese moral sensibility is folded into the aesthetic consideration of how to harmonize, and harmonize with, the real environing world. For the classical Chinese, filial family practice, political practice, ritual practice, and the practices of personal accomplishment and excellence such as T'ai-Chi Ch'uan interpenetrate on a continuum of public and private life. The practice of T'ai-Chi Ch'uan as an exercise-art is thus a personal work of harmonization that has effects throughout one's life and community. Because all art is moral art for the Chinese, the exercise-art of T'ai-Chi Ch'uan is the recreating of part of oneself as a work of art with moral force.

These high-minded considerations of Eastern and Western aesthetic sensibilities should not mislead us into pompous exaggeration of the claims of T'ai-Chi Ch'uan, as Ms Delza warns so frequently. One should not groove on the Tao when playing T'ai-Chi Ch'uan but concentrate on moving correctly and settling the mind perfectly in the movement. Forget spiritual ecstasies and just try not to fall over. The perfect movement will capture your thoughts and set them at ease. It will center the attention and tune the emotions to respond correctly to appropriate objects. T'ai-Chi Ch'uan will not bulk up your muscles but will give you the strength and flexibility to act harmoniously with the forces of your life's environment. It will not give you mystic visions but only clarity and flexibility of spirit. A little proficiency will amaze your Western friends and amuse your Chinese ones; much proficiency will baffle the Westerners and make the Chinese proud. But in all cases of taking pleasure in the responses of others, the ego can distract attention from the movement and you are in danger of tipping over. T'ai-Chi Ch'uan should be played for its own sake; it then gets better and better and its effects spread far beyond itself.

I had the pleasure of introducing Sophia Delza in a fore-word to her 1985 *T'ai-Chi Ch'uan: Body and Mind in Harmony*. There I pointed out her accomplishments as a dancer, a per-former in Chinese Theater, and a player of T'ai-Chi Ch'uan. I cited her breadth of publications, many of which are reprinted here or revised for this volume. Now I want to focus on her skill as a teacher, with special reference to her most modestly gifted student, myself.

One day in 1973 I was sitting next to William Bales, then dean of the School of Dance at the State University of New York College at Purchase, through an apparently intermi-nable meeting. I asked him *sotto voce* whether he had any dance courses that could help an out-of-shape person in his mid-thirties endure such meetings. Looking me over, he sadly shook his head No, but said the best T'ai-Chi Ch'uan teacher in the Western world was teaching at Purchase and that she would give me a "philosophical exercise." So I went to Sophia Delza's evening class just once and knew that my life had taken a new direction. After two semesters in the Purchase classes, I began attending her intermediate and advanced classes at Carnegie Hall, where I studied at least once a week for twelve years. You might well ask why it took me so long. Most people learn much faster than I. The answer is that my out-of-shape body also had no grace or natural ability and that for the longest time I couldn't tell where my elbows were except by looking. I doubt that Ms Delza ever had a student with such difficulty who didn't give up. I presented her with more wrong ways to move than she had ever seen before. But she didn't give up either, and for twelve years she corrected my form, my movement, and my spirit, until finally I got it right. During a sabbatical I went to her studio an extra day a week to watch her teach, and then taught T'ai-Chi Ch'uan myself for ten years at the State University of New York at Stony Brook. I sent my better students to her for advanced study, and she continued to teach me through them.

I am especially grateful for this book of essays and poems because they are the distillations of a long career of transcendently good teaching. Teaching too is an exercise-art that harmonizes, and harmonizes with, its environment of students. Many, many students of Sophia Delza join me in gratitude.

Robert Cummings Neville
Boston
December 1994

Notes

1. For an exact description of T'ai-Chi Ch'uan, with detailed instructions, diagrams, and photographs for the practice of the Wu style of T'ai-Chi Ch'uan, see Sophia Delza's *T'ai-Chi Ch'uan: Body and Mind in Harmony: The Integration of Meaning and Method* (Albany: SUNY Press, 1985). That volume also contains a bibliography of writings in English and Chinese.

2. A beautiful book has been produced by the Zhaohua Publishing House in Beijing (no author listed) entitled *Chinese Martial Arts* (1983), which describes and illustrates many of them as arts rather than as fighting techniques.

3. The distinction between the aesthetic and ethical sensibilities is very nicely described by David Hall in his *Eros and Irony* (Albany: SUNY Press, 1982; I have discussed Hall's distinction in *The Puritan Smile* (Albany: SUNY Press, 1987).

Preface

Depending on the nature of the individual, experiences of various kinds accumulate almost from the very beginning of study of the Chinese exercise-art of T'ai-Chi Ch'uan (pronounced Tye Jee Chwan), a system of activating the body for mental, physical, and emotional well-being.

Revealed and sensed in gradual stages are the physicality and kinesthetic sensitivity of the organic body movements, accompanied by heightened perceptivity as to how mental and emotional attributes are awakened. A growing harmony of the coordination of the formed action with the personality will at first be taken for granted; but as more and more "body-mind" information develops in extent and depth, and as detailed intricacies in the composition unfold, the relationship of the objective action to the self—that of being aware of *being in* the process itself of creating harmony—becomes a vital experience, consciously appreciated, never to be lost.

It is then that curiosity arises as to what the "means"— the method and the material—can be which evokes the harmony of calmness, ease, and physical prowess at one and the same time. Such inherent interest stirs up insights as to the constructive value of the structured organizations.

The fundamental aim of this collection of selected essays is to present, in an analytical way, the causes and the means that compose and bring to life the final "effects," this intricately designed composition, where every unit is intrinsically planned,   xix where every segment possesses its own individualized balances, where the sum of every detailed moment comprises the unique content of the masterful whole.

To know the construction, grammatical or aesthetic, of a sentence is not to erase its impact and sense. To follow mentally, to be part of and recognize the intrinsic logic of how form, movement, and spirit "tally" and link all aspects of the structure—the yin-yang dynamics, the patterned positions and forms, the "spirit" of the substance, and space-time diversity—is not to shatter mind-body unity.

Knowledge of the content, varying from the down-to-earth physicality and the equilibrium of energetic outlay, to the abstract sensation of responding to the "equilibrium" of space-time formations adds to and intensifies the experience of feeling the presence of harmonious action, as well as understanding *how* it arose.

The intellectualized knowledge of the way and the why of how the body-mind elements (the machinery) integrate and function to become ingrained eventually into the bodily activity. When the vibrations of inner "knowing" permeate the system and one feels at one with oneself, newer experiences arise, enabling one to envision as a possibility further not yet revealed sensations: the more the comprehension, the more the receptivity and acknowledgment of heightened experiences.

With shallow mental concentration, however, and carelessness in rendering the minutiae of the composition as composed, the goals of T'ai-Chi Ch'uan will only barely touch the spirit, and give the physical body only enough power to exist, but not to "endure."

As a collection of concepts, these essays may be useful to anyone who can be touched by and appreciate certain philosophical principles which can be universally applied to personal needs in a variety of situations. As a useful guide for the player of T'ai-Chi Ch'uan, the ideas can be helpful to further more profound participation in the realities of the formal content; as well as to clarify the "way" to attain, without being self-conscious, xx a higher level of consciousness with calmness and containment.

Sophia Delza

Introductory Note:
As a Beginning Experience

Over the many decades since I studied with Grandmaster Ma Yueh-Liang in Shanghai and put into practice the principles of T'ai-Chi Ch'uan, it has been a profound source of inspiration for the changing patterns of everyday living; for an awareness of the mental-emotional balance necessary to function with ease; for all kinds of personal relationships; and for teaching and other creative activities—not to forget the sensation and the assurance of being kept physically healthy, by disciplined practice and being in touch with a body in total harmony with itself.

The T'ai-Chi Ch'uan experience comes from and moves in many directions, on different roads separately felt. It can be a purely physical one, such as experiencing physical security and stability from leg and pelvis strength together with the lightness of upper torso and head. It may be an agreeable feeling that comes from the flow of the forms which link one to the other with consistent ease. These are elementary and basic reactions of one who has just begun to study.

Each "bit" of attention is a path which reveals in a very gradual way different layers of what is contained in the action. One becomes sensitive to the progress of the growth of meaning through the shades and details of the intricate process; and mind and physicality dovetail comfortably.

At some advanced stage (moment) some of the roads of perception become engaged with and within each other so that the resulting feeling-sensation is one of unity and wholeness—not of differentiation. At this time, the player has reached another level (and layer) of discernment, an awareness of interconnectedness (of many elements) which appears continually attainable.

Further experience is *never not* expected. The player is awakened to every possibility, as each "trifle" of perceptivity brings to light some other phase of activity. And the "true" player will know that there is more to come even though each step of the way brings satisfaction.

The closer the relationship to T'ai-Chi Ch'uan's essence, the deeper is the understanding of how its complexity regulates the complete nature of the "self."

Those of you who are not familiar with T'ai-Chi Ch'uan, having read this far, must be asking, what *is* this T'ai-Chi Ch'uan? Give us a definition, please—a simple one!

T'ai-Chi Ch'uan is an ancient Chinese exercise-art, a system of activating the body for the simultaneous development of physical, mental, and emotional well-being. Each aspect as defined, does not exist by its individual self. Each employs the other; that is, if the body must move, the mind is there to make it work—the action reflects the mind's power of concentration. With mind centered and the physical action synchronized with the mind's "orders," there is no necessity to worry about the emotions. The feeling will be pleasant because body and mind are not in conflict.

Harmony is the result of doing and *minding* every moment of the complex variety in this *long* structure. To this is added a very special way of movement—which is flowing, continuous—connecting the subtle links of differing transitions, from the first second to the last, some twenty-five minutes later, ideally done with a clarity and calmness which, even though not planned for consciously, come of their own accord in an unruffled temperament.

These essays are concerned with aspects of experiences which arise out of some awakening situation while one practices.

Layers of feeling or physical accuracy or mind and heart calmness may dart into the player's mind, who might find a word for
the sensations—this means that T'ai-Chi Ch'uan is beginning to
reveal itself inch by inch on a higher level of perceptivity.

We hope that the reader can "succumb" to the spirit of
the ideas as elaborated in the various chapters; and that a personalized kindred spirit will blossom from working with T'ai-Chi
Ch'uan.

The T'ai-Chi Ch'uan practitioner, newly learning or
mature and experienced, may recognize many of the ideas analyzed, may be aroused to a fresh point of view, may be completely creative, releasing *new* perceptions and "ingredients," or
may reasonably adjust in mental/spiritual/physical terms to some
of its concepts.

I naturally hope that the player will absorb the diverse
thoughts—philosophical, aesthetic, physiological—as part of the
spirit of T'ai-Chi Ch'uan's universal quality; that he/she will
have some inner experience with the "heart" of T'ai-Chi Ch'uan
in relation to the harmony of one's SELF and will continue to do
so "endlessly"—since the ending is a new beginning on a much
higher level.

Classified Chapters

The Classified Sections are so organized that the grouped essays will arouse a mental-wave of correspondence among them in thought, feelings and concepts.

T'ai-Chi Ch'uan is an integrated Art-Exercise, the Body-Mind condition of which makes simultaneous harmony of *all* the individual elements as arranged in these Sections. However, the reader may wish that one or another of them had been placed in a different category—but that is certainly valid: for example, an idea that is included under *The Tangible Spirit* may, in another context, rationally fit under *The Ever Present Substance*. The interrelationships are interchangeable because T'ai-Chi Ch'uan is a unity of multiplicities.

The classification as prepared may stimulate the mind and the comprehension of the T'ai-Chi Ch'uan player as well as, I hope, those who, though ignorant of the presence of T'ai-Chi Ch'uan, can relate and apply certain perceptions to other disciplines of thought, action and daily living.

CHAPTER I

THE CENTERED MIND

Soft and smooth, slow in time, needful
Of man's needs and nature's laws.
An art-in-movement T'ai-Chi Ch'uan
Creates a being integrated
With itself—an active, thinking,
Feeling man, engenders heart-mind
Ease, develops wondrous stamina
Beyond the age of ordinary
Retrogression and decay
      The exercise evolves, centered, quiet,
      With mind-awareness animating
      All the body's actions—from patterns
      Simple and symmetrical to complex
      Weaving of relationships in
      Intricate variety. Forms arise.
      Taking shape with myriad subtleties
      Each instant balanced and secure
            A unity of multiplicities.

The Centered Mind

1. The Mind Must Be Willing

The mind must be willing to enact the structure of T'ai-Chi Ch'uan in order to achieve a feeling of equanimity and ease. If the mind is reluctant, it is due to an emotional state (of mind) and the result will be half-heartedly experienced and un-unified.

To appreciate and to begin to understand the process of the movement and the progress of the developing forms, it is necessary to accept this fact—that the mind must be present at all times of the physical activity. To keep the mind alert and present, the determination to do so—exercising the will—is essential. This is the nature of T'ai-Chi Ch'uan discipline. The mind of the player must be willing to be brought to the stage of willingness, to participate in the action continually. When the mind is *not* willing, then we can say there is *no* exercising.

Though the structure of T'ai-Chi Ch'uan is intriguing, it nevertheless is a mental challenge to move arms and legs in differing varying formations or to go from one place to another, since there are *many* aspects which involve and demand attention. The one which is supremely necessary to attend to is that of coordination—never simple even on an elementary level. The mind that is aware of the coordinated and changing situations can function fully—even without an effort of will in some cases. All the elements of T'ai-Chi Ch'uan composition *employ* the mind.

The progress of the mind retentiveness keeps in step with the body's ability to function with increasing complexities of space-form-time dynamics. The balanced way of mind and body channels the spirit (the feelings) *away* from negative emotions as well as creating heart-ease and composure. Nothing can be done without the *mind's* instigation. Even from the beginning, one realizes that the exercise is physically based and mentally directed. With deeper perception, it also can be seen that the exercise is physically directed and mentally based.

T'ai-Chi Ch'uan, it is to be remembered, is a "from the mind" exercise for physical, emotional, and mental well-being. There is nothing in the complex structure of T'ai-Chi Ch'uan that cannot be done by the natural human body. But it is the mind that must be willing to induce the body to remain on the road to self-development.

Since the physiological laws of nature are embodied in T'ai-Chi Ch'uan, the entire exercise is objective and impersonal, not colored by individualized sentiment or background. And so it can become, paradoxically, a personal, life-long activity for all people who have "willing minds."

2. The Mind-Body Connection

The mind-body connection of T'ai-Chi Ch'uan's harmony implies that the mind is functioning at all times as the body enacts the multi-varied material of the exercise. What takes place simultaneously is what the mind imparted to the body.

In addition to being "there" as a presence, the mind must be "willing" to stay with the subject at hand. The mind trains itself not to abandon the established sequential orders to be made visible by body action: no wandering or turning itself "off," that is, blanking out. When such lapses do occur, the action of the body becomes partially automatic—for only a short time—repeating what has already been done. Fortunately, the automatic action, short-lived, "interrupts" itself and the mind is stirred to return (to itself). The newly awakened mind then makes added effort to *remain* and stay with the moment-to-moment action. By so doing, with this added awareness, the mind becomes strengthened, and as time goes on, is less likely to fade out during the long exercise. Such mind-developing education is one of the many processes—actually the *leading* one in the composition-making of T'ai-Chi Ch'uan. Without mind, none of the following features could be enacted: the subtlety of the slower motion under the basic tempo; the organization of the space and shapes; the coordinated unity of the interbalancing forms, and so on.

As the structure becomes clearer through experience, the player develops sensitivity to every passing moment of detailed movements to a greater and greater degree. The ability to perceive

8 develops with proficiency. Mindfulness—un-forced attention—accompanies awareness and recognition that a mind-body connection creates a unity that can be felt physically.

The willing mind becomes a natural, spontaneous part of behavior, and it almost goes without saying that the means and the ends are one.

3. Mind-Alert

The mind is always "there," quietly present—this is the premise (and the promise) of this body-mind exercise-art of T'ai-Chi Ch'uan. The "from the mind" concept as the inspiration for the harmoniously structured composition exists from the very first moment the beginning position is taken with awareness and endures to the very last touch of stillness at the end of the exercise.

If the total organization of the exercise incorporates mind-attention, what then is mind-alert? It suggests that in the process of performing or learning this long exercise, there will be occasions when the mind will be alerted if, for some reason or other—emotional interference, wandering thoughts, outer disturbing impressions—it has absented itself from the activity. The body, then, at such times will make a gross mistake in the pattern or sequence, and fortunately by so doing will unwittingly "awaken" the mind. That is one kind of "alert," but is not intrinsic to T'ai-Chi Ch'uan's structure.

The nature of the structure is such that its formations are so designed that in a sense they seem to anticipate a possible lapse of attention. This concept is brilliantly clear, both psychologically and technically, in the subtly astute units of transitory movements and in the changing diversity of the 108 Forms. This essay explicitly analyzes where, when and how the physical and structural "differences" have been created to keep the mind from straying.

The many technical methods, created to keep the mind steadily alert, are distinct and richly varied and are also surprising (in intricate ways). Since they are diversified, they rarely repeat the same series of patterns, never, however, deviating from the harmonious essence, but instead adding to it, aesthetically, philosophically, and physiologically. The essential qualities lie in the choreographed details that are added to or changed from an already known combination: certain units will always seem a "surprise" as if to shock one out of complacency.

The regular, organic process of sequential movements follows through without added mental pressure, flowing, connected in space-time relationships with no undue effort of body or mind, except of course for the tasks of coordination and physical stamina. The movement connectiveness of organization is intrinsic, and the player seems to move and take in the form with quiet mind and spirit. In order to prevent the mind and body from automatically expecting and accepting this steady, easy, and agreeable flow, the facts of inattention and automatic behavior already suggested above, will appear at unexpected times and are often missed at first.

We are concerned in this essay with those moments of special activity when the mind must act with greater agility, when the player becomes sensitive to an unusual state of mind, when it has "evaporated" for a second or has settled in a groove of habit.

The following analysis of a few places in T'ai-Chi Ch'uan's structure, though necessarily limited, will, I hope, illuminate the understanding of the player and prove how far beyond the ordinary T'ai-Chi Ch'uan is as a powerful subject of thought and action, mind and spirit.

How the Structure Alerts the Mind

It is to be understood that the analysis that follows merely skims the surface of the profoundly varied ways the structure manipulates the mind's attention at crucial times.

I. The Element of "Surprise" units come after a serene flow of movements which, feeling familiar, tend to become automatic.

1. The placement of the Hand Strums the Lute Form (left side) arrives early in T'ai-Chi Ch'uan structure as a surprise after a similar Form has already been done on the right side, with just enough changes (leg stance, for instance) to make the person attentive.

2. Variations of tempo are added to the basic tempo which is always "present" as done by "some" part of the body (as by a single hand movement).

   (a) *Quickened tempo.* After about eleven minutes, during which time the basic tempo is easily kept, the placement of the entire body changes with a single speedy action. Mind must prepare itself to do this, as well as to be alert to resume the basic tempo in the gesture immediately following. In Wu style, there are nine incidents of speedy action, each totally different from the others; and they never seem to arrive expectantly, the ninth being the most difficult in the final series.

   (b) *Slowed-up tempos in coordination with the basic tempo.* In the third series (Wu style), a position to be achieved requires that one arm move in a large arc, and the other in a smaller one. The basic tempo is kept in the larger space; the slowed-up tempo (relative to its size) in the smaller arc; the arms finish the Form simultaneously. This indeed takes concentration of a special kind.

   (c) *Similar Forms arriving by way of different transitions.* The Parry Form appears in the first and third series (Wu style). The transitions which connect each to the preceding formation are totally dissimilar, alerting mind to a different place and space in the evolution of the structure's mental development.

II. Repetition of Long Sequences of Forms and Transitions.

1. In the fifth series (Wu style), a passage of twenty-one Forms and Transitions which has already appeared in the second series (twelve minutes earlier) is to be repeated exactly. The player can become less centered when familiar Form follows familiar Form for a comparatively long period of time, almost moving automatically, and is therefore apt to miss the subtle point of change. The ingrained process of being with oneself, no matter how customary the action is, is part of T'ai-Chi Ch'uan's philosophy of the diversity of mind-presence. The connections of the composition are "astute" in ways to stimulate attention and awareness, whatever the occasion. This example is but one of many. The player, as a result, is accustomed to being "woken up," and so learns to stay awake, whether mind is lightly present (Yin) or deeply involved (Yang).

2. Structure also alerts the mind when Forms and Transitions are repeated in different directions. The fourth series can be a perfect tangle of confusion because the "Parting the Wild Horse's Mane" Form and the "Angel Works at the Shuttle" Form are repeated in the eight direction-changes. Actually, this series is the high point of consciousness and mind-presence. It is interesting to note here that, even after decades of T'ai-Chi Ch'uan practice, if there is a mistake to be made, it will occur in the fourth series. Coming as it does after 15 to 18 minutes of action, the player is often soothed by the flow of repeated Forms and, unless aware and attentive, will succumb to the motion of the Forms and so will miss the significant changes in direction.

III. Repeated Basic Forms Leading into Different Forms with Changing Transitions Each Time.

1. The Single Whip Form appears nine times (Wu style), six of which connect with different Forms. The mind is

alerted to a new situation, the transitions of which give the clue to the next Form. It is almost more difficult to remember the repeated connections than to follow through to the new ones.

2. High Pat the Horse Form appears five times, two of which lead to new formations during the last (sixth) series. In this case, the mind is alerted to the subtle new changes, which cannot be taken for granted.

IV. Basic Form Which Follows a Different Transition Several Times.

1. Grasping the Bird's Tail Form appears seven times, in six of which the transition connecting it to a preceding Form are different. This Form always leads to the Single Whip. This moving Form itself always has different details in its structure as it moves from place to place. This Form is a high point in the symbolism of the spirit of T'ai-Chi Ch'uan, and therefore requires "more mind."

This outline, meager in terms of what T'ai-Chi Ch'uan contains, will perhaps suffice to illustrate the play of mind—how essential it is to use the mind to enhance perceptiveness, to develop quick reflexes of thought and action.

David Darling says in his enticing book, *Equations of Eternity*: "Nature's strength is in the physical, Man's strength is in his Mind."

T'ai-Chi Ch'uan's structural harmony is in its physical strength (nature), and in the strength of man's mind.

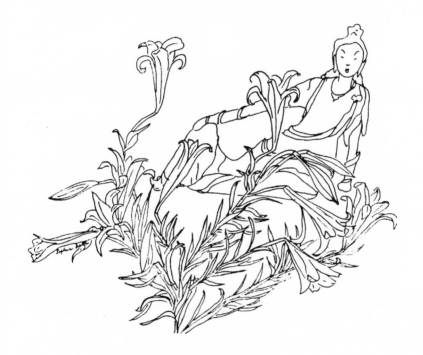

Equanimity

4. The Unifying Principles

The thought of self-exercise seems to arouse two negative reactions in the Westerner—the first, that it is a thoroughly boring business, and the other, that one exercises to slim down. Too often I am asked no question other than whether this or that movement will make one thin. The thought of developing strength, stamina, suppleness, or flexibility, never arises nor does the idea of improving the circulation, to mention only some of the *physical* reasons for exercising. It rarely occurs to people that there is also an emotional aspect connected to correct movement, or that the mind, too, must be engaged and stimulated in order to feel truly and agreeably well.

Actually, most people underestimate themselves. When they find exercising boring, they are really looking for something to interest their minds and, although they are not aware of it, they are unconsciously criticizing the nature of the exercise to which they have been exposed—repetitious, unvaried movements which do not have enough complexity to arouse and sustain interest, and which soon become automatic and are done without thinking. Boredom sets in when the heart and mind are not engaged.

A Philosophy

In the Chinese exercise-art of T'ai-Chi Ch'uan, the approach to exercise is completely different, the opposite of what is described above. It is a *philosophy* of body-action, a total exercise, so called because it incorporates a way of making the mind direct the action and a technique that stabilizes the emotions while exercising the complete physical body externally and internally.

It was in Beijing that I first saw this exercise in action, at dawn in the T'ai Mizo park. Dozens of people, young and old, were each doing his exercise, each clearly centered on himself. No outside sound of voice or instrument directed the movement. The slow, continuous flow of form and the impeccably even tempo seemed to come not only from some mastery within each one but also from the intrinsic nature of the action itself. Complex patterns followed one after the other in an unimpeded sequence. There appeared to be a variety of unrepeated designs which balanced themselves at every fraction of a second. It was as if gravity did not exist. Looking amazingly light and stable at the same time, each person's movements seemed effortless. It was apparent that a distinct and formal structure existed, with every movement a clear consequence of what had preceded.

This was indeed a fresh experience for me. I soon realized that it was not dance that I was seeing, although the elements were those contained in a dance-art. As a dancer myself, I could see the designed body and space structure and the movement quality that are significant in any fine body-movement art. What gradually became clear to me was that the *intention* inherent in the exercise—the spirit, the psychic energy, the psychological attitude—differed from that of any performing art, directed as the latter art is to the spectator, who is the recipient of the content of the dance-expression. In this case, no audience was needed, although to me, looking in on it, there was no doubt that a spirit of containment emanated from the action, however unintended. The "doer" was the sole recipient of the beneficial content—emotional, physical, mental, and spiritual—from what I came to know as "T'ai-Chi Ch'uan."

Awareness

The distinctiveness of T'ai-Chi Ch'uan as an exercise lies in the mastery of the *material* of the body—thought, feeling, and physical mechanisms. The integration and harmonious relationship of these centers—body, mind, and emotion—frees the personality and makes possible further development of awareness and a higher level of consciousness with the awakening of latent faculties.

Although it is centered on the self, it is not self-centered, not narcissistic. It does not isolate one from the world of activity and thought; ethical teachings of Chinese philosophy pervade all aspects of art, culture, and self-development techniques. Through the application of the principles of T'ai-Chi Ch'uan, one becomes more adept at handling one's experiences and environment with the equanimity of a stable disposition and an alert mind, lasting effects from the persevering practice of this exercise.

Appreciating these concepts of T'ai-Chi Ch'uan will not and cannot construct the visual picture of its Forms any more than knowing the values and qualities of a musical composition can make us hear it. Nevertheless, because T'ai-Chi Ch'uan is a way of believing, as well as a philosophy of behavior incorporated into a system of activating the body, it is not misleading to speak of its content. We should, however, never forget that "true knowledge originates in *direct* experience," since T'ai-Chi Ch'uan is not an intellectual exercise.

Book of References

T'ai-Chi Ch'uan did not emerge full blown out of one man's mind. It took hundreds of centuries to become what in the Ming dynasty (fourteenth century C.E.) was considered a complete entity, unified in structure and philosophy. At this time the *T'ai-Chi Ch'uan Ching* (Classic) was formulated, which has been and is today the vital manual of this ancient art.

Back of it were the constructive thought and experiments of ancient philosophers (fourth century B.C.E. Taoists) and the thinking and practices that developed in the ensuing centuries—thinking and practices designed to promote a sound body and an attentive mind. It involved an ethical attitude aimed at bringing about a more "realized" man.

T'ai-Chi Ch'uan had its early inspiration in the T'ang dynasty (c. seventh century C.E.), beginning as a slow, continuous, calming exercise called Ch'ang Ch'uan (Long Ch'uan). It took six hundred years or so more until Chang San-feng, called the "Father of T'ai-Chi Ch'uan," finally created its "universal" Forms. This took thirty years of concentrated effort in developing a comprehension of "the way of man" in relation to "the way of nature."

What the basic philosophy of T'ai-Chi Ch'uan is, which has been so well established over the ages, and which pervades Chinese thought, conduct, art, can merely be hinted at in an explanation of what T'ai-Chi and Ch'uan is.

Yin and Yang

T'ai-Chi is a concept of mutuality, comprised of two balanced "opposite and complementary" vital forces: the principle of duality which when in action "makes the world go round" and gives rise to the "10,000 things" (everything in the universe). The two vital reality energies are called *yin* and *yang*, and are in continuous movement. To give a few examples—in yin-yang order, they represent, night-day, moon-sun, cold-hot, negative-positive, female-male, space-time, square-circle, empty-solid, close-open, dark-bright, and so on.

The essence of T'ai-Chi is visualized by a symbolic "diagram" of a circle divided by a reverse S waveline into two spaces, the shadowed side being yin, the bright side yang. A light dot in yin and a dark dot in yang indicate that there is a perpetual interchange between the forces, and that one cannot exist without the other. The embracing circle holds the continuum of action in balanced wholeness and adds stillness to movement.

Ch'uan is literally a fist, metaphorically implying control, containment, defense of the self, as well as nonaggressive power, an exercise for activating the body for physical, emotional, and mental well-being. T'ai-Chi Ch'uan is then a Ch'uan according to the way of the T'ai-Chi, conforming to the spirit of duality with its ever-moving alternating changes in form and dynamics. (There are hundreds of different Ch'uan exercises *not* related to T'ai-Chi in the immense repertory of Chinese exercise styles.)

Balance

Constructed in yin-yang terms—shape, structure, space, time, movement, stillness, and activity—each and all are intricately related in a complexity of ways, yet remain in perfect balance with respect to the two forces. Even the outer appearance and the inner feelings are complementary opposites, the outer look being airy, light, thoughtless, while the inner force is solid, firm, concentrated, and strong in its dynamic tension variations.

With its 108 *Forms* (yin) and 108 connecting *transitions* (yang), T'ai-Chi Ch'uan is an ever-changing process (yang) where an ending is a beginning, which, in turn, leads to an ending, a repeating cycle, repeating.

Change is mentally manipulated for the dynamics of form, architecture, positions, patterns, time, and spacial directions. Change is essence—and being the "matter" of the moment, it can be said to generate itself. Obviously, change without a point of reference, a focus, would be chaotic and destructive. The invariable unity of yin-yang balance in each and every differing part in T'ai-Chi Ch'uan is the central core, the axis, a changeless oneness, ever present, like the North Star in the heavens.

Continuity

One of the many ingredients of the T'ai-Chi Ch'uan composition, of the greatest importance to me, is that of continuity—the fact that the exercise does not stop, halt, or rest at any point in its execution. Once begun, it continues in a movement line I call seamless, for 22 to 25 minutes. Although the motion moves forward and back, in and out, expands and folds back on itself, it progresses smoothly and evenly as "pulling silk out of a cocoon," to put it in the words of the *T'ai-Chi Ch'uan Ching*.

You might well ask: (1) Doesn't one feel exhausted, wearied, fatigued by keeping up such controlled activity?

(2) Wouldn't one feel breathless and have a quickened heart-beat? (3) With such ceaseless motion, doesn't one become bored and irritated? (4) Isn't the mind pretty well overworked at having to direct the body without an instant's rest? Answers to all of these questions are contained in the principles that lie at the heart of this unique exercise.

Vitality

The answer to the first question is that freshness and vitality result from doing this exercise, never exhaustion, despite its length and ceaselessness. The designed patterns are so devised that different parts of the body, at different times, have the burden, so called, of the action—one part is rested by using yin or light dynamics, while another part is activated with strength; or one part is still while another part moves, all alternating in a scientifically ordered sequence of changes. The process of this changing continuity on which the mind is centered creates endurance and profound vitality.

Yin-yang works without conscious exertion. Energy is never expended through superfluous and needless intensities. One learns to use only the amount of effort required by the act. All the Forms in the exercise are given only that amount of force "built in" to the movement. Thus, when the total body functions with minimal effort, then clearly it is not being drained of strength, and not being drained, stamina can be accumulated and stored up. We can therefore say that energy is used productively. To be able to behave in this way is to keep the body in untaxed equanimity.

Energy is kept from "seeping out" and "being employed extraneously by the circular, arcing, and spherical nature of the gestures and the curving path of the movement as it goes from place to place in space. A circle is "an urge to wholeness" (V. Dyson); a curve, an arc, a wave or spiral engenders a feeling of containment, lightness, and ease.

Positions, forms, transition-connectives constantly alternate with differing degrees of complexity and simplicity, which prevents a situation from arising that would become overpowering and, therefore, fatiguing.

To sum up, with the structure of ever-changing Forms and the variety of dynamics in unremitting play, with energy used intrinsically, naturally, and with physiological consistency, not even the *thought* of weariness and exhaustion can arise!

Effect on Heart

As for the effect on the heart, T'ai-Chi Ch'uan is a slow, soft-intrinsic exercise. No demands are made on the heart as is required in swift action. The tempo in which it is done is in tune with the rhythm and speed of a healthy heartbeat. It therefore moves in that functioning tempo, slowly and because of the intrinsic, flowing nature of the slow movement, the resultant look is "soft," light, and buoyant. "Soft" does not mean slack or weak. It is like the softness of water, which while appearing so, is in reality powerful, resilient, and sure. With such a soft and slow movement, there is no possibility of quickened breathing or heart action. Moving in this contained way creates poise, patience, and power.

With respect to boredom, the orchestrated composition of the 108 Forms is so complex and has such variety that there is always some new experience, some hitherto unperceived subtlety, to spark the interest and awaken awareness, even after years of practice. The surprises in the variegated themes, the intricacies of coordination, the appreciation of the dynamic changes in relation to space-form, are persistently present—all of which keep the mind wholly engaged, and as it directs all the action, there is little chance for boredom to set in. In itself, the technique of the flowing, connected, light, and soft movement calms the spirit and cannot ever irritate it. Neither mind nor body ever "sleep-walk," that is, remove themselves from the presence of the activity and behave automatically. When the mind is interested in what is being experienced then life has meaning, and with meaning, how can one be bored?

With such insistence on presence of mind, with every induce-
ment to keep it alert, awake, and involved, the question of its
becoming overworked is indeed apropos, this is *not* the case if we
remember the principle of T'ai-Chi and its cyclic course of change.
The mind, too, is affected by the philosophy of change and is
sensitized to varying shades of effort and release, of deep concentrated activity and restful repose.

These opposite forces are put into play by the demands
of the forms in terms of strength and power, by problems in
complexity, by familiarity of theme, and by the length of the
unit of structure. At strategic moments some Forms are repeated
to alleviate the intensity of the mind's effort, after which released point a complexity in a new Form will arise requiring a
greater degree of concentration to direct the multiple action.

The pressure on the mind's activity is greater for a complicated situation, obviously, than for an elementary one. When
greater physical effort must be made, such as in the act of standing on one leg while at the same time intricate movements are
being made by arms, hands, and trunk, the mind and body are
fully engaged, but soon an easier combination will follow to
"soothe" the mind.

The mind and body stay together like shadow and substance, synchronizing their activities to the minutest shade, producing ease and contentment.

Unified Action

The characteristics I have thus far enumerated and analyzed to
allay the fears aroused by the thought of a long continuity of
action, are also integral to T'ai-Chi Ch'uan as a whole. There is
no one feature isolated from the other; they all are interrelated.
Every Form is a complex aggregate of unified action.

In addition to these features, intrinsic to the essence of
T'ai-Chi Ch'uan are the concepts of *balance* (physical, mental, and
emotional), *totality* (the body as an organic unity), and *silence* (activity executed without sound accompaniment).

The adjustment of the mental-physical, spacial-dynamic
forces of the body into a unity of stabilized equilibrium can be
termed *balance*. Physical balance related to gravity is essentially
the result of the mathematical structure of T'ai-Chi Ch'uan,
which distributes weight, space-time, form, and dynamics in perfect proportion. So subtly and minutely are the forms and the
transitive connections created that centered equilibrium exists
at every point and *second* of this long exercise.

Mental Balance

The control of body-movement organized by such an infallible
structure creates emotional and mental balance. The necessity
to concentrate and direct the body in order to execute the form
exactly and correctly, develops strength of mind and prevents
the mind from straying. The mind, being centered, is balanced,
and balance is a unity of action and thought. Action-thought
unity creates feeling (a heart) which is not erratic or restless.
Balance is a harmonized wholeness.

The symbol of T'ai-Chi (described above) represents the
Great Balance where every cause is an effect and every effect a
cause. T'ai-Chi Ch'uan is a unity within space and time and if
stopped at any point of its unfolding evolution it still would be
in perfect physical (structural) and yin-yang (philosophical)
balance.

The physical, emotional, and mental aspects function
simultaneously and mutually benefit each other. At every moment in every movement there exists a totality that is never
diminished, lost or separated. This is even apparent in the experience of a beginning student who must concentrate on the
"what to do" and is not yet cognizant of what goes into the
making of the "*way* to do"; even he/she, despite the elementary
nature of the disciplines, experiences a special kind of peaceful
satisfaction, a glowing calmness from the activity, although the
essence is not yet mentally comprehended. The personality di-
gests—so to speak—objective elements and appreciates them
subjectively.

T'ai-Chi Ch'uan is without ego since action is not inspired by temperament and self-expression (Gaiety, sadness, etc.). No personal interpretations color the Forms with free associations, as in children's play. Concepts are philosophical, psychological, poetical, moral-ethical, metaphysical, and, for some, mystical.

108 Forms

The names of the 108 Forms are each symbolic and signify concepts removed from the literal physicality of the object—horse, tiger, bird, and so forth. Each name has its separate allusion, and metaphorically may connote an aspiration, a philosophical attitude toward self and conduct, a turn of mind, a sense of being, some thought about life and spirit. The true meanings are revealed when the T'ai-Chi Ch'uan exponent has advanced to that stage of experience comprehension where he can utilize the implication of the philosophical intentions, and where the symbols can be part of his growing consciousness. This happens only when the mind and body have "changed" and absorbed the reasons for mental, emotional, and physical unity.

With profound and prolonged practice, the exercise becomes "second nature," and can be done easily and seemingly spontaneously. But no matter what the Form and action are, the mind's presence is indispensable.

To be lost in thoughts is to be truly lost when doing T'ai-Chi Ch'uan, for then the automatic mechanism of the body will take over and make one lose one's way. The structure fortunately is such that it is impossible to continue any sequence "blindly asleep" for more than a few seconds. An error will be made because the body-system will, out of habit, revert to a former pattern sequence, which will then jar the mind awake. The statement that "Habit is a great deadness" (Samuel Beckett) is definitely proved when we experience a situation where a habit-gesture (action without mind) has destroyed the form and killed the awareness—even for a moment.

The mind propelling the Form and the Form instigating the mind to aliveness exemplify the reciprocal interchange of yin-yang, in this instance mind (yang) affecting the Form (yin) and vice versa. The pleasurable advantage is in the fact that there is no separation of mind and body, from which totality everything seems "to come out right." As Chang Chung-Yuan says, "It is unification which achieves harmony."

I wish to elaborate on the extent to which the mind is present, having used the phrase "presence of mind" so often. When one knows T'ai-Chi Ch'uan thoroughly, even to the degree of understanding structure in terms of "space-self" and appreciating its most subtle intangibles, you might ask, fairly enough, whether the mind has still to be a "presence."

The Mind Process

There are different layers or levels to the mind process. In the learning stage the outer mind sends the messages and directs the thought or action. The inner mind, having accumulated the knowledge, "knows" and reacts speedily—a lightning flash between plan and execution, thought and act. Training and experience develop quick reflexes, but only if there has been close concentration in the repetition of the act. When the mind works well, it is *as if* the "inner" mind weren't there, *as if* there were no mind movement.

To illustrate the instantaneous performance of mind and body, let us take the example of stepping off a curb. We note the curb and the mind prepares the body for a change in movement, all *as if* it were happening without the mind's being involved, so immediate is the reaction, and at the same time thoughts or conversation have continued without interruption. It appears *as if* we were reacting without thinking, but how well we know the uncomfortable shock our body gets when we do *not* anticipate the curb because our mind message has not been sent.

And so it is with the exercise in all its multiple changes of weights and measures. Eventually, with experience, the inner mind takes over. Centered, it sees and does all in the right place, at the right time, for the right reason. This could not be accomplished without concentration. Just as the eye focusing on a given point can see everything within the periphery of its vision, so the mind, knowing and centered, can propel the coordinated action like a complex musical chord in one synchronized split-second. Perhaps we can say that when one begins to understand "with" the body and the inner mind is ready with its accumulated knowledge, then the magnetic force of T'ai-Chi Ch'uan is "doing" us. When this occurs, then one has indeed reached a high level of development.

Organic movement is the method by which the body's changing activities are made to function with great economy of effort. The structural range of patterns, designs, postures, and so forth, is determined by the logic of physiological laws in the control of the pull of gravity, for the purpose of remaining in perfect equilibrium at all times, as well as to prevent one from being immobilized by its force.

Wholeness

The balance of strong-light dynamics and the complementary play of opposites in every moving line and combination are the source and the consequence of impeccable physical balance. The entire body acts with such complete unity that even in a very detailed and refined movement combination, a wholeness exists. In T'ai-Chi Ch'uan, form and function are an organic entity.

I have already noted that T'ai-Chi Ch'uan is performed, practiced, "played," as the Chinese put it, in complete silence: no sound of drum; no musical phrase to lean upon, to divert, or inspire; no voice to direct the tempo or animate the expression. There is nothing except one's self to take one out of one's self. One is in total command of one's self. With such self-dependence

is developed a true experience of movement relationships with
the intrinsic necessity of activity and form.

Silence

The mind can concentrate on the moment and the *pre*-moment
to prepare itself for subsequent action without cues from outside.
The mind makes one self-sufficient in the silence of the act. In
silence the mind can reject extraneous thoughts and can prod
itself to be present when it has wandered. Silence helps one
remember oneself, through which one reaches to a higher plane
of consciousness.

Quiet is essential for awareness and attentiveness—to
hear oneself from inside out, and so be able to call up to the
surface of the mind deep-seated thoughts revealing an anxiety, a
wish, a fact, a hope, which rises like a flash, pertinent and significant. With experience and control, silence helps to limit the
mind to the subject at hand and the interference of irrelevant
ideas diminishes with progressive experience. Just as the physical
body (chemical, dynamic, mechanical) gradually acquires stamina,
ease, and proficiency, so the ability to dissolve the flood of
thoughts, which are destructive, progresses with experience, too.
Being silent is far from being heavy or leaden. On the contrary,
it is pleasurable and tranquil. Since it is beneficial, we can say
that silence, in more ways than one, is golden.

T'ai-Chi Ch'uan is a lifelong exercise for a good long
life, since physically it corrects and improves the health of the
body in all aspects internally and externally; emotionally it relaxes the nervous temperament, "gives one a good disposition,"
and, "by ridding one of arrogance and conceit" (Ma Yueh-Liang's
and Wu Chien-Ch'uan's *T'ai-Chi Ch'uan Manual*), produces
calmness and serenity. Stability profoundly increases alertness
and awareness necessary for "human faculties to display all their
resources . . . enlightened by reason and sustained by knowledge"
(*I-Ching*).

A mark of pure poise and self-control is the ability to
move in multiple ways quietly, with the correct dynamics, with

power and lightness, easily, gracefully, and calmly. The outer appearance is always light and stable in repose and activity; the equation is balanced ease. The power to act with such harmony is due to the nature of T'ai-Chi Ch'uan itself, which is a philosophy of action and which puts into action a philosophy for the continual development of the self to a higher level of health and consciousness.

5. What Gives a System Validity?

Many years ago I was taught by grandmaster Ma Yueh-Liang in China that there are various systems or schools of T'ai-Chi Ch'uan—Chen, Yang, Wu, Sun, Ho—each stemming from the previous one, and all coming from Chang San-feng's original way.

Today there are many styles, which are modified, changed, cut, diminished, expanded, and so on. They are styles but not necessarily systems.

What makes a "style" legitimate as a system?

Throughout the 1,000 years since Chang San-feng created the concept, it is clear that T'ai-Chi Ch'uan has changed as it passed from master to master. It has changed in structure, but not, it must be emphasized, in principle or goals.

If the principles which are the heart of T'ai-Chi Ch'uan are kept truly intact, then doubtless the style is legitimate. It is kept intact not by "word" message alone but by the fact of the inevitable rendition of the physiological laws of nature and the philosophy that arises from the harmony of change on every complex integrated level of the structure.

Deterioration sets in when Forms are eliminated and connected arbitrarily, when there is thoughtless and careless rendering of structural relationships, when changes are motivated by personal whim and subjective wishes.

A newcomer to T'ai-Chi Ch'uan will render the Forms inefficiently, but experience and knowledge plus diligence will lead to improvements. If the basic principles are taught and embedded into the analysis of the technique, the student will more easily perceive the heart and meaning of the exercise.

When teachers do not deal with time-space dependencies and omit the aspect of stillness-in-action and fail to distinguish the subtleties, T'ai-Chi Ch'uan becomes action without depth or variety and therefore becomes a deteriorated version.

Deviation, however, can be legitimate when changes come from philosophic understanding of the totality of T'ai-Chi Ch'uan. The changes over the centuries from Chen to Yang, Wu to Sun and Ho, have been scientifically created and spiritually based. The masters of each perceived fresh nuances with differentiations of arc, curve, and balance on a foundation of physiology and philosophy.

These systems conform to the harmony of structure, keeping body and mind as one unity. When the changes are in perfect balance at every instant and yin-yang principles are kept clear, then the system can be considered to be "legitimate."

That one system has "more" to it than another—such as subtleties in "time-form and space"—is of the deepest significance: it is that one master has seen more intricacies than another, and has extended the physical and mental image.

My interpretation of the Wu system (which I practice) is that the "eye and mind" have discovered and made visible certain situations that were *already* ingrained in T'ai-Chi Ch'uan but had as yet not been exposed.

Let me explain it in this way: an astronomer discovers a "new" star in the heavens. Obviously, it was always there. But it was not visible to man's eye or the previously available telescope. With a more developed instrument (eye) and increasing knowledge (mind), the scientist "discovers" what has existed.

In a similar fashion, a master of T'ai-Chi Ch'uan with his deeply developed knowledge and experience, more subtly attuned to the essence of T'ai-Chi Ch'uan, discovers or discerns further subtleties in T'ai-Chi Ch'uan structure which had been present but hitherto were not felt, seen, or analyzed.

T'ai-Chi Ch'uan, with such new awareness, becomes richer in substance and spirit. The greater its multiplicities, the more profound is the *experience* of the unity of mind and body.

CHAPTER II

THE TANGIBLE SPIRIT

The body moves itself around in
Space, in many figured forms, young in
Legs, mature in mind, the spirit bright,
A harmony in structure and in
Quality. The balances of Yin
And Yang, like shadow and its light
Are poised: though opposite, are friendly
And compatible, both constantly in
Motion, interchanging equally
   Gathering and separating,
   In-out-low-high solid-void, concrete
   And intangible, stillness and
   Activity, airiness and weightedness
   Molding all in varying degrees
   Of intensities, the seeds of one
   Come to a fruitful finish which
   Itself becomes a new beginning
     Endlessly unending.

34

The Tangible Spirit

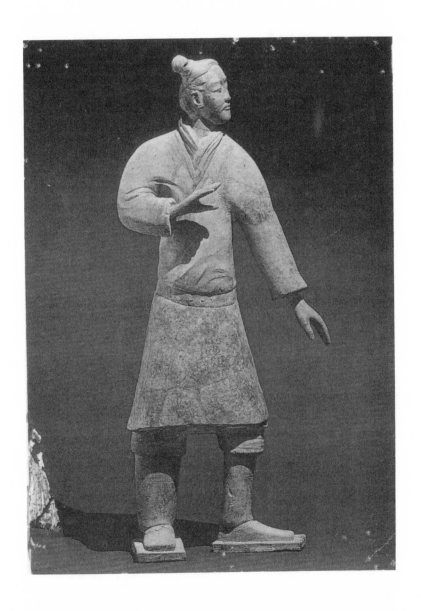

Alert Attention

1. The Moving Spirit

As we move along in flowing style through the forms of T'ai-Chi Ch'uan, a special sensation is unfailingly present—a pleasant feeling of repose that seems to make a unit of body, mind, and emotion. This feeling-sensation, which coexists with and corresponds to the activity that is taking place, can be called "The Moving Spirit."

The simultaneity of moving and spirit is so uniquely achieved in this exercise-art that we need hardly ask whether it is the spirit that moves or whether it is the movement which gives rise to the spirit. One blended with the other, with cause an effect and effect a cause, creates a wholeness which contains the spirit of the moving.

The outer body (muscles-joints-limbs in space-direction-placement) and the inner mind (awareness-attention-perception) are always in touch with each other. With the ever-present structural harmony, the movements shape the developing patterns into significant Form, without which there can be no spirit. The continuous manipulation of the Forms with concentration and consciousness contains and releases a spirit of calm well-being and alert equanimity. To be aware of self and to sense selfless objectivity while in space-time balanced movement is to capture and to experience the Moving Spirit.

From the very first movement of T'ai-Chi Ch'uan, the mind's presence and the control of a constant continuum urge the spirit to emerge or make the spirit come to life. The body as a physical force, the body as a psychological entity, the mind as the ever-present power, all merge harmoniously, philosophically and practically. This integrated harmony constitutes the spirit and is the spirit-centered calm, aware and concentrated.

Even from the very beginning of one's study, at which time form and movement can hardly be understood fully and which certainly cannot be performed correctly, even then, the process of moving in the T'ai-Chi Ch'uan "Way," with multiple patterns and balanced dynamics, stirs up a new feeling that is more than physical. It is a "spirit" inherent in the nature of T'ai-Chi Ch'uan (and all great art) that touches and envelops even the raw beginner. When comprehension develops in depth and with relative accuracy in rendering the structure, then clearly the quality of the feeling-sensation becomes richer, more subtle, and profound.

In essence, T'ai-Chi Ch'uan is a composite of the art of activity which unites the personality into a totality, the physical self being involved with the mind, the mind stimulating the body, and both together affecting the emotional condition and the spiritual aspect. Functioning physically in the prescribed way with its harmonious complexities and united energies, T'ai-Chi Ch'uan will reveal the nature of the Moving Spirit and the presence of the spirit moving.

Since "that which transforms the form is the spirit" (Binyon, *The Flight of the Dragons*), at the completion of the exercise, with the finishing touch of the final gesture, the feeling-sensation does not disappear. Though the outer activity has ceased, the inner activity goes on. The Moving Spirit penetrates the system for several seconds, and this length of time is increased as one's experience moves one to a higher level of awareness and technique.

Many of us have felt that delicious calm that settles over us when we give ourselves in unselfconscious relaxation to the setting sun and the light of twilight. At that hour, nature creates an almost total stillness, even though the subtle changes in shades of color and shapes of clouds are steadily intermingling.

This feeling is not the kind of calm that comes from T'ai-Chi Ch'uan, where the calm is of our *own* making, and accompanies the Moving Spirit. Whereas we react to and accept the sunset's quieting affect, with T'ai-Chi Ch'uan we create the quiet through our *willed* activity by recreating harmony. Calm is within us and spreads outwardly, never fading but gradually augmenting with use and self-growth.

The calmness of sunset touches us from the outside inward, and although we respond most agreeably to it, it does not have the power to change us from inside out, except temporarily. The sunset's calm has a settling effect, we become *be-calmed*. But T'ai-Chi Ch'uan produces the opposite result; we acquire an enlivening, *vital* calm which the Moving Spirit promises to make permanent.

2. The Eloquence of Silence

T'ai-Chi Ch'uan speaks for itself in the exquisite smoothness of its activity, in the quiet flow of its dynamic movement, and in the lyricism of its tempo.

Awareness of the paths of moving, concentration on the way of movement, produce a magnetic vibration which makes the lack of sound go unnoticed. Not heard but felt, the inner voice of T'ai-Chi Ch'uan speaks out, is sensed (though not quite understood) by anyone who comes within the visible field of its activity.

Unprepared as I was for T'ai-Chi Ch'uan when first I saw it in Beijing, I responded to it as if it spoke out to me personally. The unaccompanied movement in structured balances projected a quiescence not only as if "aural," but also emotional, and I felt a magnetism which seemed to send forth meaning and essence.

T'ai-Chi Ch'uan needs no outside influence of sound accompaniment to lean on, to interpret, or to speak for it. We can say that it sings out and fills the air with an orchestrated composition which has a resonance that amplifies itself with structured variations of spaced time, phrased themes, and with subtly textured inner/outer harmonies. In "concert," all project a quiet which is distinctly heard.

This quiet speaks to us as does the silent dawn, which is not at all like the deep silence of midnight nor like the stillness of fading twilight. Dawn-quiet is fresh and bright and seems to promise a new awakening.

So T'ai-Chi Ch'uan resumed each day acquires new clarity, develops depth of insight as to what we can say to ourselves as we "listen" to it.

With the external silence of T'ai-Chi Ch'uan which helps to make the mind less noisy, with quiet attention and calm spirit, we can hear the inner voice of T'ai-Chi Ch'uan make its meaning become more and more resoundingly clear. As time goes on and experiences accumulate, T'ai-Chi Ch'uan and its way of silence vibrate more eloquently.

3. With an Air of Innocence

T'ai-Chi Ch'uan is an innocent-looking exercise. Yet how can we use the word "innocent" for such a complex mind-body structure, so philosophically and aesthetically profound, a structure which scientifically integrates space and form and balances mind concentration with intricacies of body activity?

T'ai-Chi Ch'uan has the appearance of innocence because it is a continuum of flowing movement without any visible change of dynamics or tempo. Being in unfailing balance at all times adds to the look of ease and, therefore, the air of innocence.

Since in T'ai-Chi Ch'uan no emotion colors the activity and no intellectualizing interferes with the making of the forms, all action appears to grow naturally. Anyone who experiences the exercise will always feel "just right," whether the person is mature or fairly new in the practice of this exercise-art.

We do not say it is an exercise *for* the innocent. It can be learned by the most sophisticated, by the naive, by the very ignorant. The exercise is simply done step by step with mind directing the manner of movement and the matter of patterns, from which the participant will feel its harmonious objectivity.

T'ai-Chi Ch'uan is as "innocent" as breathing—without which we cannot live and yet which we accept so innocently and matter-of-factly. T'ai-Chi Ch'uan functions for all— naturally—because it is organically consistent with the laws of nature and permits us to behave with the physical regularity of breathing.

The unified balance of the whole makes the inner experience joyous and profound and, with it, produces, outwardly, an air of innocence.

Experiencing T'ai-Chi Ch'uan is more than a matter of balance, continuity, and concentration. In the final analysis, it is the greatness of the harmonious structure which vibrates with meaning and which insures the containment of innocence.

From the first moment of action to the last moment of stillness, the meaningful structure puts the T'ai-Chi Ch'uanist into a state of aware receptivity. The presence of the mind in the activity of the body, with the body alert to the activity of the mind, produces a look of "no-thought."

Through the unity inherent in the many complexities, T'ai-Chi Ch'uan itself, *not* so innocently, creates a situation in which the participant cannot but project an air of artlessness and so seems innocent.

4. Spontaneity: The Look of Ease

Spontaneity in doing T'ai-Chi Ch'uan comes after long, repeated practice of the entire exercise. When all is ingrained in the system and is mentally directed, only then does T'ai-Chi Ch'uan activity have the effect of being performed with spontaneity—as if with no thought and no mind.

Spontaneity arises not only from the feeling of familiarity and the accomplishment of every detail spatially and physiologically, but also *especially* from deep comprehension of the spirit of the whole.

If one is to appear spontaneous and to experience ease, no awkward movements, no extrinsic forcing, no mechanical rendering of patterns and positions are possible or permissible. No emotional or temperamental moods may color the action. These all would disrupt the inner process of ease—ease which is the ultimate quality leading the way toward spontaneity.

It is commonly thought that a spontaneous art springs from the heart without any thought interference—out of nowhere into the light of day. A sudden decision to behave in a certain way is often termed spontaneous. But the cause for action may have been embedded in the mind for some time, awaiting the propitious moment to be put into external action.

This is *not* the spontaneity of T'ai-Chi Ch'uan. An example of what occurs in T'ai-Chi Ch'uan, where the effect is spontaneous, when the content and technique have been thoroughly studied, is that of the performing pianist whose trained fingers glide over the keyboard perfectly with all the expressive nuances seemingly executed without any thought. Only after years of practice, acquiring technical skills and understanding of musical essence, can the pianist produce, without effort, the atmosphere of spontaneity.

The same approach applies to the T'ai-Chi Ch'uanist. When every aspect has been learned excellently, the entire exercise becomes so much a part of the person that T'ai-Chi Ch'uan appears to be unstudied. Then, it truly has the look, the easy look, of spontaneity—almost as if it were being improvised freely.

Being in complete *control* at all times—which means recognizing and conforming to the principles of the philosophy and structure of the activity—constitutes the essence of spontaneity. For instance, when one is writing and the words move smoothly along the page, the brain and the hand are simultaneously in control. The letter, the word, and the concepts emanate from knowledge, and it is knowledge in any activity that gives control. Therefore the act of writing, flowing unhesitatingly, seems free but is actually controlled by knowledge, with mind centered and aware.

In T'ai-Chi Ch'uan, one senses a feeling of satisfaction in being in control of oneself in relation to the exercise and in being in control of the exercise in terms of one's self. One feels free and at ease in experiencing the exercise as being under one's control.

Such freedom is framed by knowledge—being sure of all aspects of T'ai-Chi Ch'uan with mind in control. The appearance is that of spontaneity, the inner feeling is that of freedom, secure and easy.

Because of the innate harmony of all elements in the structure of T'ai-Chi Ch'uan, this exercise cannot but produce an organically organized reaction—that of being in total balance. With the development of increasing knowledge and control, both freedom and spontaneity ensue progressively. The look of ease, the air of spontaneity will arise inevitably, and T'ai-Chi Ch'uan, to quote grand master Ma Yueh-liang in Shanghai, will become "second nature."

5. The Student Is Forever; Learning Is Forever

Is it a discouraging or an optimistic thought that the student is forever? It would be quite depressing if the student remained forever on the same level of meager knowledge or even on an advanced level. It would also be depressing if the student did not see the possibility for further growth or did not perceive that there was more to know. When the goals are recognized as being profound and when the technique, though complex, is enticing as well, the idea that learning is forever is invigorating.

To know is to want to know more, which indicates that there is more to know . . . an ever-satisfying progress. However, it would be frustrating to contemplate "forever" as a perpetual state if each "knowing" point were not itself an agreeable whole, a completeness that radiates quiet pleasure and which leads to another more searching experience. This is the promise of T'ai-Chi Ch'uan at all moments.

Just as the artist always feels himself or herself to be on the road to greater creativity, just as the inventor moves ahead after fulfilling an idea which in turn may be the seed of another thought, so the student—at any level—is perpetually moving ahead in depth, in physical stamina, in mental discernment of the objective exercise, and in the more subtle awareness of self and, especially, of some unique harmonious experience within.

To repeat, T'ai-Chi Ch'uan as a physical exercise *only* is impossible. It is impossible because of the intrinsicality of this exercise. All the elements co-exist and are revealed at the very same moment of the action. These seep into the system of even the most ignorant and eventually reach conscious levels of awareness.

To do is to know and to know is to do more and more with ever-increasing ease and sensitivity. But being a student does not always imply the presence of a teacher-in-command. Being able to be a student by oneself, of and for oneself, proves the vital and constant growth in thinking, feeling, and doing of a more highly developed person.

No matter how great the master teacher is (or was), the furthering of knowledge and experience becomes a matter for self-penetration and illumination. Only from such self-progress can comprehension arise which further illumines the entire subject of T'ai-Chi Ch'uan as a balance of harmonious change. The perception of the material and the immaterial of T'ai-Chi Ch'uan continues to develop in the "forever student" under his/her own masterful eye and mind.

And when the student becomes a master on other levels of comprehension, he/she is, nevertheless, a student experiencing, perceiving, and developing forever, in form and spirit.

6. The Ending Is a New Beginning

At the completion of T'ai-Chi Ch'uan, having made a "full circle" with awareness, a singular sense of harmony is experienced.

Spacially and physically, the patterned Forms have traveled in many directions, touching at different times all points of the compass in a 360° circle. This fact, in itself, is not the only reason for the awakened feeling of fulfillment. It is due to the total composition: (1) to the curvilinear nature of the continuous movement; (2) to the minutely harmonious relationship of "all" that is taking place; (3) to the presence of the mind at one with body-action.

The "full circle" is physically, psychologically the expression of body-mind-space-time structured-harmony, all coordinated to a fraction of a minute. The moment of the "ending" is a stay of action alerting one to the stillness within one—a feeling akin to what is felt at the beginning but with a difference. The stillness at the ending contains the essence of containment on a very deep level. The beginning stillness is mentally made; the ending stillness, having grown intrinsically in the process of experiencing the structure as a whole, pervades the entire being—the emotions, the body, and the mind

The action of T'ai-Chi Ch'uan, having traversed a large world of space and shape, finally arrives at the position (bodily and spacially) in which the exercise began. Though externally similar as are the body stances at the beginning and the ending, the spirit, *however*, at the ending is very different—obviously—since the T'ai-Chi Ch'uanist has moved through a world of harmonious changes and is hardly the *same* as when he/she began.

What is extremely interesting is the developing keenness of consciousness as one moves through the ever-changing harmonies of the multiple forms.

At the close, all complexities of action disappear to become a simple unit of movement, as was the original stance.

Physically and mentally, the two stances are hardly the same: the *start* opens to awaken the yin and yang dynamic; the *finish* is "neutral," containing no feeling of differentiation in the torso or legs. All is light (nonmoving), as if magically suspended.

Whereas the attention at the start is poised for action, the mind at the end is centered in stillness.

At every stage of "advancement" in rendering T'ai-Chi Ch'uan, a more profound element is generated which makes the ending more gratifying and elated.

Whatever the final sensation is, a comfortable calmness lingers on intrinsically for a long time after moving away from T'ai-Chi Ch'uan's final moment.

When T'ai-Chi Ch'uan is resumed (on another day), it is always on a more elevated level of awareness. Each repetition advances to yet another stage, to open up deeper and more subtle insights; the ending is then a very new beginning.

CHAPTER III

THE EVER-PRESENT SUBSTANCE

Feet firmly in control of gravity,
Head and arms float and soar, all
Weightless as in stratosphere
In supple action joints are joined
Like wave to wavelet on a quiet sea.
Muscles move in flexion and release
As easily as flower-petals
Open-close for light and night
Yielding to necessity
      Ease produced from strength unseen
      So gliding ducks seem effortless
      Their forceful motion hidden
      From the surface of the water
      Outer calm and inner power
      Lightness and stability
      Agility and energy
      Co-exist in T'ai-Chi Ch'uan
         A magical duality.

50

The Ever-Present Substance

1. Landscape of the Self in Action

We accept the fact that all the component parts of the T'ai-Chi Ch'uan structure are put into harmony by the organic relationship of different parts of the body's moving structure. What characteristics do we see in the way various parts of our bodies act in terms of the principles and qualities destined to be achieved by the T'ai-Chi Ch'uanist?

Do we know the way each part is manipulated and how each contributes to the unity of the whole? Can we understand how all work together to make a "landscape of self" beautiful, comfortable, and integrated?

Each part, I have found from my analysis of intrinsic form and action, can be individualized as to the fundamental quality manifested by its "behavior" in making a gesture, in going to and arriving at a position.

It seems to me, and it pleases me to think, that the following attributes can be considered to be significantly basic to each designated part in the landscape of the self. I hasten to say, however, that some qualities can be "reassigned," as it were, to other parts with good reason and psychological coherence. The following are the different parts of the body and their individual qualities.

> Head—Steady
>
> Face—Imperturbable

Eyes—Eloquent

Neck—Secure

Shoulders—Unemotional

Arms—Impersonal

Hands—Intelligent

Torso—Knowing

Waist—Accommodating

Pelvis—Cooperative

Legs—Invincible

Spine—Assured

Fingers—Significant

Feet—Responsive

Elbows and Knees—Willing

Wrists and Ankles—Acquiescent

All are mindful. Note I have not used characteristics which the entire person possesses, such as calm, patient, aware, alert, controlled, flexible, pliable, concentrated. These are aspects of T'ai-Chi Ch'uan as a whole. Altogether, all succeed in creating tranquillity, stamina, ease, and containment.

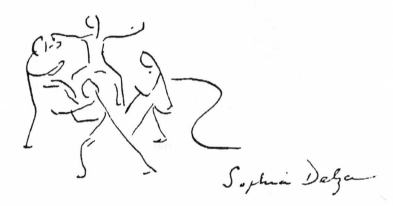

Attentive Stillness

2. The Long Journey

T'ai-Chi Ch'uan takes you on a long journey. It is a long and smooth journey, a long and integrated journey; above all, it is a profound journey. This slow-in-tempo journey can make time disappear. Sometimes it seems endless; or it may pass like a grand and monumental moment; but the journey itself will always move you with clock-time accuracy.

The journey is a complex one. The extraordinary paths of diverse movements are *never* not in balance and *never* without coherence and unity. No matter how subtle the action and intricate the maneuverings, the body-journey structures are physically at ease, and fall exactly into place in space and time, three-dimensionally sculptured.

As a profound journey, it is never abandoned by the mind, which not only directs the action but keeps you attentively aware and clear. The stumbling-blocks of entangling emotions, distracting thoughts, and mental blank-outs are erased as the journey progresses.

A hyperbole of balance, the journey functions securely in physical-emotional-mental dimensions.

T'ai-Chi Ch'uan, at each stage of its journey, fulfills the varied, promised goals directed toward a higher development of the self in terms of keener consciousness.

As a process of change and a changing process, nothing in the journey is trivial, nothing superfluous—from the most solid tangibles to the illusive intangibles; from the minute turn of a wrist to the augmented power of a stance; from a complex element culminating in a Form to the simplicity of an isolated gesture. Always throughout, the dynamic forces, light and strong (yin and yang) interweaving, are sensitively graded.

The journey creates many experiences and awakens awareness on many levels—physically, psychologically, intellectually, artistically, psychoanalytically, creatively. These aspects may overlap and be enmeshed one into the other or may be discerned separately. Always pleasurably interesting, every step of the way offers satisfaction for body and mind and for the spirit—even very early in the journey.

The greater the development, the more assured become the will and the willingness to repeat and continue the journey which inevitably becomes richer, more subtle, and more powerful. Although the journey in terms of self-development is endless, it has an ending in time, at which point the activity—the outer activity—ceases physically. All visible motion then has come to rest, but the journey within the self continues—consciousness of being calm, awareness of the presence of a quiet yet alert self, of a newer vitality.

This journey's end becomes a new beginning, since every repetition contains the advanced and accumulated experiences of all that went before. We can respect the ever-increasing power of mind and body that each journey produces. Once the journey has been undertaken, the feeling that there is no end is extremely agreeable. As self-knowledge augments, it is intriguing to anticipate what could possibly happen as the *inner* journey progresses in depth and self-confidence.

When we say that this journey is "out of this world," we imply that the journey is more than could have possibly been perceived at the early stages of moving on the T'ai-Chi Ch'uan path. As one travels far enough, consciously enough, and *often* enough, the resulting unusual and contained sensation can be considered to *be* "out of this world."

Though it is important to get to the end of the journey for full effect, it nevertheless offers rewards at a succession of the "smaller endings." Each of the 108 Forms is a definite culmination of shorter sections and passages of varying time-lengths. These are the many "stations" of awareness on the way as one travels toward the end.

During the journey, there is no feeling of division or separation. The totality—the sum of the "small journeys"—brings one to a high level of accomplishment at every repetition of the entire journey.

T'ai-Chi Ch'uan, stronger than the self, helps one to enture the journey as it becomes progressively more profound.

3. The Harmonious Anatomy

As I use the word *anatomy* in connection with T'ai-Chi Ch'uan, it is more than the physicality of body-action required by this exercise, more than the manipulation of muscles and joints to form positions in properly balanced relationships, more than the technique to control the continuity of the sequential movements of the composition.

Chinese artists and philosophers, in discussing the aesthetics of the art of painting, believe that a painting is more than its "flesh and bones" (that is, design techniques). The Chinese expression for this *'more'* is *Ch'i-Yün*. Oswald Siren, in his book *The Chinese on the Art of Painting*, translates Ch'i-Yün as *"spirit-resonance."* It is the vibration of vitality and a "resonant" spirit which calms the heart and "excites" the mind. *Ch'i* is the life-force, the "energy of everything"; *Yün* is resonance.

T'ai-Chi Ch'uan, too, is more than its designed composition and technique—its "flesh and bones." The anatomy of T'ai-Chi Ch'uan, to be truly harmonious, must possess the essence of Ch'i-Yün, which will arouse in the T'ai-Chi Ch'uan player vitality, calmness, and mental alertness.

It may well be asked, where does the spirit-resonance come from—what produces the vibration of vitality—what is the quality which "excites the mind," that is, gives it perceptivity, and at the same time the feeling of calm and quiet? Are those sensations continually present; are they being gradually developed; are they felt only at the completion of the exercise?

The harmonious totality of the complex structure of this exercise-art is of such profundity that even a beginning student-player cannot but experience a dimension of feeling-awareness beyond that of physicality, a feeling which is a combination of energy and ease—which arises without conscious intention, without planning or anticipation.

Similar feelings could not possibly be evoked by any other type of exercise, however agreeable. Only a richly organized exercise such as T'ai-Chi Ch'uan, based on universal organic principles, the mathematical balance of forces and space-time relationships of dynamics, can affect the mind, body, and spirit simultaneously.

The 108 Forms and the equal number of transitions (as in the classic Wu style of T'ai-Chi Ch'uan) are integrated by the dynamic interchange of yin and yang. These energies relate to the physical aspect of movement and form, as well as to the angle of direction of all the positions taken in space.

Fundamental to the complete structure is the variety of the continually changing configurations and combinations of body-action, all kept in perfect balance by a coordination of movement which is spatially timed.

Since one of the high aims to be reached is that of longevity, it stands to reason that emotional stability and mental alertness play clear and definite roles in the consideration of what "health" means.

Personal Anatomy, Objective Anatomy

The three centers of the human system—the physical, emotional, and the mental—mutually sustain each other. Interlinked, they comprise what I term the *personal anatomy* of T'ai-Chi Ch'uan for which the structured composition has been created. Every part of the body, from the most minute to the largest, is activated at some time or other by the complexities of the method and the way the structural elements work. The design and techniques—that is, the "flesh and bones"—which put T'ai-Chi Ch'uan into action, form its *objective anatomy*. One of its essential qualities is the intrinsic way of moving, uniquely different from the extrinsic way. When the body exerts no more effort than what is needed by a particular movement to put it into action, the movement is called "intrinsic"—built into the body-way, done without any emotional interference.

To illustrate: Standing on one leg places the entire weight of the body on it, making its muscles behave with super strength. When two feet are on the ground and share the weight, each leg then "uses" less muscle power, an obvious example of the intrinsic behavior of the body. A raised arm uses more energy than does a hanging relaxed one. A flexed wrist necessarily puts the arm muscles into play. These simple gestures exemplify the natural "built into the body" way, the muscular effort changing because of placement and movement form.

This applies to every action in the T'ai-Chi Ch'uan complex structure—each one of which provides the proper amount of effort and energy to be expended—with no emotion accompanying or prodding the gestures to make a greater-than-needed effort.

Because the movements, from place to place, can be made in a light (intrinsic), flowingly even, continuous, and "balanced" fashion, they do not reveal the inner (felt) dynamic variations. To the viewer's eyes, all appears to be equally "soft"— with no trace of stress. T'ai-Chi Ch'uan is called the "soft-intrinsic" exercise (as I learned it in China), differentiated from "tensed-extrinsic" exercises. Soft, directed outwardly, is what the observer sees; firm, functioning inwardly, is how the player feels.

The structure of the composition as an organization of 108 Forms and Transitions includes:

1. The aspect of moving continuously with no halting or stopping, no matter how "complete" the forms, taking a minimum of 25 minutes to perform in perfect basic tempo.

2. Balanced interweaving of the yin-yang dynamic alternation.

3. Coordinative exactness in manipulating the designs in space and time.

4. Precision in placing, in correct relationship, in the floor-space so that at the completion of the exercise, the position ends exactly where it had been begun.

These are some of the outer aspects of the objective anatomy—mathematical and physiological—which the player attempts to render exactly. The personal anatomy, physically and mentally, becomes transformed by the uniquely integrated harmony of the objective anatomy features; here nothing, no fraction of a movement, is expendable.

Tempo contributes to stability; coordination to serenity; diversity to concentration; the intrinsic way eliminates stress and strain and gives ease and energy. All together, functioning simultaneously, they awaken the possibility of the development of spirit-resonance.

Absorbed as we can become in the structure of the objective anatomy, we nevertheless recognize that it is the *mind* of the personal anatomy that determines the eventual development and the maturing of the "spirit-resonance." It is the centered mind which points the way and permits us to live alertly and consciously. Without mind there is little action beyond the instinctual. In China I was taught that T'ai-Chi Ch'uan is a "from the mind" exercise, and so it was *always* called.

Mind directs every fraction of the body's activity as it moves in and through the amazing intricacies of the structure. Mind tells the body what to do; the body knows intrinsically how to do the action properly according to the physiological laws of nature. The mind significantly is the basic and the ultimate means which makes the "blending" of the personal and objective possible. Mind is the measure of their harmonious existence. Such unity, when sustained, awakens in the T'ai-Chi Ch'uan player patience, calmness, and ease, vitality and alertness. An awareness of a special kind of feeling, the nature of which gradually leads to the perception of what is to be attained eventually (with years of practice), touches the player at all times, at no matter what stage of competence.

When the player and the "form" become inseparable, acting as one, it can be said that negative emotions and stray thoughts have been completely eliminated; and it is then that the player will truly experience equanimity, the most desirable essence residing within the harmonious anatomy of T'ai-Chi Ch'uan.

It is pertinent to return to the early reference of Ch'i-Yün, the spirit-resonance, which a great work of art possesses and which term I have applied to the exercise-art of T'ai-Chi Ch'uan.

There is a decided difference between the way Ch'i-Yün works for T'ai-Chi Ch'uan and how it works in and for the art of painting.

The finished painting, the picture itself, carries the message, the meaning of which illuminates the viewer, who experiences it with mind and emotion. The artist has expressed himself, and with his art hopes to awaken a deep response, the awareness of Ch'i-Yün, in those who can absorb themselves in the art-aesthetic.

Whatever T'ai-Chi Ch'uan "offers" is for the player alone, for each player individually recreates the established choreography. That person will, by the very doing of the exercise, give life to its spirit, both in becoming the "medium," so to speak, and by being the "other half"—the personal anatomy of the objective anatomy. No observer, on seeing T'ai-Chi Ch'uan as it is being performed, can feel more than agreeably moved by the fluid action; he can only wonder at what could possibly be felt by the player, its spirit-resonance will never touch him.

From the steady concentration displayed by the player, the observer can surmise that something "special" is being experienced other than the pleasant physicality of the exercise movement. What *it* is can never be perceived or faintly guessed at without oneself actually participating in the complexities of the exercise itself. The player and the observer are worlds apart.

Yet, the inner worlds of the T'ai-Chi Ch'uan player and the art-viewer who is immersed in the art and the heart of a great painting reach and touch a similar chord of feeling. Both share, comprehend, and respond to a profound spirit deep within; that resonance which enriches the total being by stimulating and expanding the life of the mind, by nourishing a sense of calmness, and by "lifting" one's spirits.

These enlivening effects, in response to a great work of art-painting, are short-lived for the beholder, since they do not imply a way for him to apply them to the conditions of everyday life.

For the T'ai-Chi Ch'uan player who lives in and with the harmony of the exercise, all aspects of the practical and philosophical aims become ingrained in his/her personality and behavior; to be calm is to act calmly; to have vitality enables one to function well at all times mentally and physically; to become increasingly perceptive makes one rise to higher levels of development—beneficial to society as well as to self.

Spirit-resonance, the integrated quality of the whole, is as "concrete" a part of T'ai-Chi Ch'uan as is each and every separate element of the structured choreography. It is this all-pervading essence which makes the anatomy of T'ai-Chi Ch'uan harmonious.

4. What Is the Nature of "Soft"?

The word soft may imply weakness, flabbiness, inertia, and lack of energy. It may be thought of as overripe and overwilling, and it may stand for flexibility, pliancy, and resiliency—which is exactly what the "soft" of T'ai-Chi Ch'uan means, especially when it is united with "intrinsic."

The intrinsic nature of T'ai-Chi Ch'uan gives the word soft its special quality, being the very opposite of hardness, tightness, rigidity, inflexibility. We cannot but *appear* soft when we move intrinsically, when we permit the body to use its own sense as to how much effort is needed to perform a particular act, then we are moving and arriving at form intrinsically.

As examples of the "built-in" soft-intrinsic nature of movement, it is natural for the legs to use more muscular strength when activated than it is for any arm movement in whatever direction. It is natural for the pelvis and hips to function with more dynamic force than is necessary for the torso to adjust itself. The flexion of the foot will "automatically" energize the lower leg. A hand bent at the wrist will stir up tension in the arms. All dynamics are internally motivated.

Such intrinsic behavior is ever present in every turn of movement, however small, and in all changes of the complex T'ai-Chi Ch'uan composition. The degree of dynamic differs more or less for every movement, depending on space, proportion, tempo, and the process of moving connectives.

What is the effect of this? The *appearance looks* soft and effortless. But *all* is effort and control, nevertheless. "Soft" is the result of impeccable balance, the lack of strain in manipulating gravity, and the perfected combinations in coordination. . . . All together, they make effort seem nonexistent. Thus, the T'ai-Chi Ch'uanist will give the impression of effortlessness and total softness, this outer appearance being the very opposite of the firmness, strength, and "minding" taking place within the body.

Understanding the intrinsic, built-in inevitability of form and function, the player can eventually enact them correctly, and act naturally enough to permit the *body* to do the task of making the range of movements properly dynamic. This is "soft."

The sensitive T'ai-Chi Ch'uanist appreciates the yin-yang nature of the body—the upper part from the waist up being light, the lower half having the "burden" of the weight of the whole body, and which therefore must behave with greater power.

When each part balances the other, then the totality appears light, soft, flexible, and mobile. And when the entire body feels *secure*, then the feeling of lightness with the look of softness prevails.

Soft-intrinsic is a single thought which makes the inner power and outer lightness simultaneous at all times.

5. The Integrated Exercise

T'ai-Chi Ch'uan is a system for activating the body for the simultaneous development of physical, emotional, and mental well-being. It is useful for the actor because it promotes a heightened perceptivity, sensitivity, and stamina. Since the exercise has no stylistic mannerisms, it enhances the ability to manipulate the body expressively for any desired effect.

T'ai-Chi Ch'uan has a long history. Its roots go back into the Chou dynasty (fifth century B.C.E.), when concern for physical and mental health was being expressed in a philosophy of movement. But the organized exercise of T'ai-Chi Ch'uan as we know it today dates from the twelfth century. It has evolved from the philosophical concept that the mind and body affect each other to the mutual advantage of each; that to increase the ability to concentrate and coordinate is to raise both mental and bodily powers; that equanimity (heart-mind ease) must be part of, and the result of, the exercise-action.

What relevance can this ancient exercise have for the actor's craft? What are the ingredients of action, thought, and structure that can develop a superior technique that is physically important for the actor as a person and a performer? What are the ingredients that can lead to a mastery of self and a spirit that imbues his work with imagination, variety, energy, perception, endurance, and subtlety? These are not such formidable questions if we consider what strengths—in terms of body, mind, and emotion—are needed to play any given role. A good, well-functioning body is not enough; it must be an "understanding" one that can respond readily to an idea or a situation with flexibility, sensitivity, profundity, and assurance. The actor must be capable of a wide range of expressive "textures," and he must be in control of body changes and adjustments. In short, he must have a mind that is quick to perceive, responding with swiftness and clarity both to himself and others.

The practice and knowledge of T'ai-Chi Ch'uan, one way or another, can have an effect on every aspect of the mind and body that the actor needs to call upon for his role.

One begins the exercise in a position of *utmost ease*. Eventually, the practitioner learns to move and perform complex body arrangements with the utmost ease. How does one start with this feeling and yet have to learn to do it and be it? Well, the ability to function with a minimum of effort for a maximum effect is what the technique of this exercise is all about. The technique of T'ai-Chi Ch'uan can be found in its science and its art. It is the art of structure and form (personal and special), which functions with the science of body structure. This body structure is knowing what to do and how *not* to do, of moving so organically that one can be in tune with the mind as well as with the action.

Essentially, T'ai-Chi Ch'uan is a philosophy of body development, which is concerned with function and form. It produces emotional stability almost as a spinoff through the harmony of thought and action achieved as a result of practicing the exercise. The body is activated through a wide variety of predetermined arrangements, where the mind instigates the "doing" and the act of doing involves the emotions. The entire structure in a utilitarian sense is controlled by a constantly shifting interplay of light-strong dynamics (yin-yang changes), much like the energy of a wave where the push and release in alternation create and become the wave. Cause and effect are one. To do this exercise is to *be* it.

T'ai-Chi Ch'uan, therefore, is a total, integrated exercise. Although "total" is a word much bandied about these days,

I do not hesitate to use it since it is intrinsically applicable to this form of body activity, embracing as it does the totality of man's being.

The simultaneous use of mind and body is where the value lies for the actor. The exercise frees the actor to become what he needs or chooses to be through the mastery of the physical body so that it can function with correct or easy energy, simultaneously making the mind concentrate. The use of the body and mind then helps to put one into a state of calmness. The actor feels "whole" and totally confident, not distracted by random thoughts and victimized by irrelevant emotions. It is this "state of well being" that acts as a tranquil base for creativity.

T'ai-Chi Ch'uan is actually a structured composition of 108 Forms, which are interconnected by an intricate variety of subtle transitions. It is done ("played" is the Chinese word for it) as a composite unit in which one moves continuously for 22 to 25 minutes. It is designed to take place in a definite space, which is related to the action of the body. There are no loose ends in this exercise. Each thread of motion flows to and joins the next with such inevitability, both physiologically and aesthetically, that it can never seem mechanical or arbitrary.

The awareness of spatial relationships and the movement quality contribute to the practitioner's feeling of satisfaction. A "settling" of the emotions is achieved by the unity of (personal) self and the (objective) environment.

T'ai-Chi Ch'uan's long time-span of sustained action is an ingredient that develops physical stamina and endurance, patience (emotional), and concentration (mental).

The variety of action calls for reaching a plateau of competence through coordination that is on a level of sensitivity as "subtle as a poet's turn." The exercise awakens comprehension of how the body functions in a multiplicity of ways and yet is in command of the complicated action that is perceived as a unified whole.

Many in the West consider an exercise as only that kind of movement which takes a strenuous, tensed effort, along with swift force, to execute. They believe that strength comes only from expending energy violently. T'ai-Chi Chuan's technique is the very opposite. The basis of its spirit and philosophy is that by *not* straining (which exhausts), by *not* forcing movement (beyond necessity), by *not* exerting strength (which strains), by *not* over-activating heart and breathing rhythms (which depletes), vitality can be stabilized, true strength increased, and energy enhanced.

The *way* of moving is the essential quality. It is slow, even, light, continuous, and in balance; each Form flows into the next without stopping. The variety of the structures puts every part of the body into play, from the smallest joint to the largest muscle. This forms patterns which pass from one part of the body to the other without overworking a single part. The alternating interplay of dynamic tensions promotes fine circulation. The scope of the tangible and intangible structural relationships keeps the body from tiring itself. The curvilinear movements (spiral, arc, parabola) contribute to the calming process, and the weaving quality of these motions prevents effort from being expended uselessly, building up a reserve of energy with potential force like "a bow about to be snapped."

Intrinsic Dynamics (Physiological, not Emotional)

The impetus for making movement strong or light, tensed or released is never inspired by personal feelings. Changes in body dynamics are caused by what the body itself does, by how the body moves, by where the body is going, by what parts of the body are moved (in combination or separately), by what holds still and what is active. The energy of muscular contraction or release comes from the "built-in" process, which is intrinsic to position, action, and spatial movement. All this is natural to the need at the moment. No thought or emotion colors the quality of the action. A basic example of such an intrinsic feeling would be to stand with both feet placed wide apart, then bend both knees as if sitting on a horse. While staying in this position, note how strong the tensions are in the thighs, ankles, feet, and buttocks. The torso should feel light. Then straighten the knees and note how much lighter the legs are. Nothing forced the muscles to change *except* the action itself.

In T'ai-Chi Ch'uan, the conscious awareness of such intrinsic dynamics is increased through the experience of "internally" directed change, rather than "externally" directed change (where the muscles react to an outside force). An example of an externally directed change would be to hold any empty kettle under a running faucet. As the kettle fills up (without touching any surface), note how the arm must flex to hold up the weighted kettle. The reaction of the muscles in this case is to an *outside* force.

T'ai-Chi Ch'uan is a soft-intrinsic exercise, where the muscles react to the "workings" of the body in an uncountable variety of changing shapes. An example of this would be to close the hand and make a light fist. Then, open your fingers slowly, spreading them apart gradually. When they are relatively straight, the fingers by themselves will, being apart, force the muscles to energize. Now let the fingers move into each other, and the muscular flow will be clearly apparent in its lightness. Then bend the fingers and close the fist, and you will find that even with a light fist the hand will feel (and be) stronger than an open hand. The meaning of the word "soft" in all of this is that the appearance of all the described action does not disclose the felt dynamics. All the movements have an even and untensed (that is, soft and floating) appearance.

With T'ai-Chi Ch'uan one learns to function intricately at many levels of awareness. Once the body can behave naturally (correctly aligned and in balance) in all of its maneuvers, then the mind can be *with* "the heart of the matter" required by one's work, undisturbed by physical problems.

Context (To Function with Form)

In T'ai-Chi Ch'uan progress is made from Form to Form. The details of each Form are practiced as part of a whole and are never taken out of context. One never moves one part of the body repeatedly as is done in other exercises, where the head, for instance, might be rolled, or the shoulders agitated, or the torso twisted over and over again. All movements in T'ai-Chi Ch'uan are interrelated, so that various units are organically built up. The body is never merely a mechanical instrument, even when the paramount concern is just adjusting joints and spine, hips and shoulders, eyes or neck. The body is brought to a higher level of functional perfection by the structure as a whole as well as by the unity of smaller units that contain all aspects of the whole, such as stillness and motion, force and nonforce, power and lightness (and shades thereof), variety in balance, a beginning and an ending. No one thing is repeated in succession. And this continuous use of sequences, distinctive and unique, stimulates the mind and keeps one from being bored. It awakens the imagination while exercising the body so that one learns to use all in context naturally.

Forms illustrate the process of integration and totality in activating various parts of the body in context with the Form. The natural changes of dynamics are determined by changing position, with stillness (yin) and action (yang) combined. The total Form is sensed as being "just right" when one gets the feeling of the impeccable balance of design-shape-movement dynamics. This feeling is especially agreeable when the mind is quietly focused.

What has this feeling of harmony of mind and body to do with the act and art of acting, directing or other activities in the field of theater? To be restrained by emotional disturbances limits the ability to create with freedom, imagination, and profundity. To put oneself into an agreeable state of mind immediately loosens tenseness, physically as well as emotionally. If T'ai-Chi Ch'uan had no more to it than to help calm stage nerves, it would be of value to the actor. Even if it were nothing more than a "physical" exercise, it would accomplish more than is usually explored in "regular" extrinsic exercises. The actor begins to "see" himself with this objective exercise. Since it is a total exercise, the "benefits" are not exclusive of one another. In T'ai-Chi Ch'uan, the actor will find that *slowness* produces patience, poise, and power; that *flowing continuity* produces perseverence, grace, and ease; that *variety and complexity* produce concentration, coordination, and quick reflexes; that *interplay of dynamic changes* produces flexibility, resilience, and assurance; that *clarity from the mind* (the opposite of automatic behavior) produces alertness, perceptivity, and personality; that *circular movement* gives security, reduces nervousness, produces calmness; and that *activity combined with stillness* produces attentiveness, control, and stamina.

The actor thus becomes an expert in handling himself through T'ai-Chi Ch'uan. He also becomes a master of tranquillity.

In closing, let me quote the definition of tranquillity from the I-Ching (Book of Changes): "Tranquillity is a kind of vigilant attention. It is when tranquillity is perfect that the human faculties display all their resources, because [then] they are enlightened by reason and sustained by knowledge."

STILL MOUNTAINS
AND
FLOWING WATER

*A time for work and a time for
rest—so man's years ripen.
In nature he*

sees (jiàn)

*the rhythmic pattern—movement
and rest.*

Mountains

now written–

MOUNTAINS 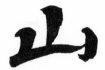 shān

*in their grandeur
and serenity,
manifest strength born of
stillness.
Lao-tse said: "Who can
make the muddy water clear?
Let it be still, and
it will clear itself."*

Opposites in Unity

Rippling water
now written–

shuǐ

WATER

in its ebb and flow, manifests
strength born of movement.
"Nothing so gentle, so
adaptable, as

water (shuǐ),

yet it can wear away that
which is hardest and strongest."
–Lao-tse.

Nature's rhythm—movement
and rest—is symbolized in every
Chinese landscape painting by

shān

mountains (shān)

and water (shuǐ)

never one without the other.
Hence–

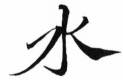

LANDSCAPE

shānshuǐ

Opposites in Unity

6. A Glimmer of Insight into the Substance of T'ai-Chi Ch'uan

We touch upon this subject with caution. Insight is profound; it is abstract; it is rich in meaning. It can be incorrectly thought of as being "knowing"; and it can be confused with attention—simply attending to one's activities. Although knowing and attending contribute to the "appearance" or the recognition of an insightful reaction, it is definitely more than either or both together.

Insight is a matter for both heart and mind. Arising as it does from awareness and experience of body-form activity, it will, in the proper course of events, reveal the meaning and the spirit of T'ai-Chi Ch'uan.

Insight into the substance of T'ai-Chi Ch'uan cannot be gained simply by knowing only the *what* of the exercise, that is, the placement of the patterns in correct physiological and structural sequence.

Of all the advanced steps in the "knowing" and doing aspect, the most important is the *how* of the exercise, that is, by what means and methods, technical and mental, the formations come into being as one form leads to the next with impeccable logic; how cause and effect balances the distribution of the elements of time-space-form-shape dynamics; and how the order of continuity progresses. Uninterrupted attention on the *how* of the *what* that is taking place is essential to the possibility of insight being aroused.

Acute awareness of how the movements unfold to create a unity of diverse elements will, in addition, contribute to the awakening of a distinct feeling of pleasure. This state of heart and mind is intrinsic to the act of "seeing into" the harmony of the specific activity. When such a sensation is enhanced by an understanding (that is, knowledge) of the complex aspects that causes it, then it can be said that that feeling has been touched by a glimmer of insight into the "workings" of T'ai-Chi Ch'uan. Awareness of what is being done as it is being done (to the very second) makes one sense the harmony—and that, in the long run, is the pleasurable reaction.

To gain insight into the nature of the "behavior" of T'ai-Chi Ch'uan, that is, the *how*, requires a developing sensitivity to the uniquely structured composition: to wit, experiencing it on a physical level; discerning the relationship of the transitions as they significantly move to and from Forms (the 108); appreciating the space-tempo coordinations; experiencing the dynamics of lightness, weightiness, and the "neutral"; knowing how the flow of movements can be so consistently continuous; detecting the coordination of the intricacies of small movements. (These are a few of the many possible experiences.)

Experience and knowledge of the above-mentioned ideas are acquired gradually, and arrive in many "installments," as it were. One grows and ascends from one stage of knowing to a more subtle one, with more penetrating perception.

It is inevitable/natural to grow within T'ai-Chi Ch'uan, because each one of the changing technical aspects feeds, adds to, and leads into other phases with intrinsic consistency—as naturally as a plant passes through various stages of growth, ultimately coming to fruition.

The following aspects point out and emphasize some of the many "state of mind" situations which, if experienced, will eventually incite further insights into the harmonious relationships of "things"; that is, the process, the form, the composition.

Awareness: of how the coordination process harmonizes space and tempo(s).

Appreciation: of the balanced interaction of form and direction, that is, the changing quality in a form facing a different direction each time it is repeated.

Feeling: the easy calm of the curvilinear movement, no matter what part of the body forms it: hands, arms, legs, feet, torso, head.

Sensing: the self, controlling the passage of flowing movement through any spaced area—tiny or large.

Distinguishing: the culminating wholeness of a Form as an ending, and as the beginning process of a transition leading to another Form.

Recognizing: how a slowed-up tempo of a small pattern coordinates with a larger one moving in basic tempo, in order to reach a specified place simultaneously.

Differentiating: the yin and yang dynamics of energy and those of space-direction.

Discerning: the totality of the Form in which certain parts of the body are held still, while other parts are moving: balance of stillness and action.

Experiencing: the significant presence of the circle-wave position as it appears in different ways: as a Form or as a movement in transition.

Concentrating: on the details of the structure, noting the smallest links in the wave of the action—subtleties of physical movements which alert the mind.

Note that any of the above descriptions can be analyzed from different points of view—all are interchangeable. We can appreciate what is sensed, differentiated, or felt; can sense what one is aware of, and so on. Each and all depend on the degree of development of the individual. No matter what the order of experiences seems to be, the final result is destined to be the same: comprehension and self-experience of the *substance* of T'ai-Chi Ch'uan—the state of mind-body-heart in harmony.

"Discovery" by oneself of the more subtle elements that compromise the connections of form-quality-placement, is a proof of deeper perceptivity and richer body-experience.

　Such growth indicates that "insight" into a particular sequence is not far behind. It may arrive (be perceived) gradually or in a flash; no matter how, where, or when, the glimpse will be supremely pleasant and the knowledge of it gratifying.

With further development in the art of T'ai-Chi Ch'uan, and with a developing keenness of insight, one feels the integrity of the *how* (method) and the *what* (composition). The unity of small parts becomes as significant as is the structure of the whole. Nothing is superfluous nor superimposed in the Form; nothing is done without essence. The action with the flow and formal structure seems to activate itself. When one is concentrated, there is unique feeling as if the exercise itself were using the body as a "medium." The person and the action are in equal and balanced equilibrium.

Suffice it to say that insight "makes itself felt" when concentration on the coordination of a varied set of movements is truly constant. Insight is never mentally urged, nor can it be self-consciously forced.

The great creators of T'ai-Chi Ch'uan had profound insights into the meaningful qualities necessary to prolong the life-span, to calm the disposition, and to enlighten the mind. They were inspired to create an external form of bodily exercise which would function as a practical means to achieve those ends, physically and spiritually. Whereas the T'ai-Chi Ch'uan master moved from "inner" philosophical concepts to create an "outer" physical form, the student of T'ai-Chi Ch'uan proceeds from the "outer" technique to progress to "inner" knowledge.

The physical-emotional-mental experience with this "external" exercise brings into existence, on various levels, insight into the substance of T'ai-Chi Ch'uan, the nature of its physical-mental harmony.

CHAPTER IV

THE BALANCED SCALE OF STRUCTURE

The outer form distils in outer air
A radiating calm, it circulates
The inner air, the Ch'i, to inner
Places "subtle as a poet's turn."
Form touches outer air at eight points
Of the compass: these "eight" with "five"
Directions, forward-backward, left-right-
Center, identify themselves with
Diverse universal elements.
      Mountain-marsh
      Heaven-earth, water-fire
      Wood and metal, earth (as matter),
      Summer-winter,
      Spring and autumn,
      A positive composite
      Greater than the self
      Thus making self
            A greater possibility

The Balanced Scale of Structure

I. A Miracle of Movement

In an airy, sunlit studio at Ohio University in Athens, I had just begun a demonstration of T'ai-Chi Ch'uan when, as someone later told me, a butterfly alighted on my shoulder and remained there for fully fifteen minutes—till the moment when I had to change the slow, flowing tempo to a flash of speedy action.

Lao Tzu wrote, "When the harmony of yin and yang is perfect, a bird can sit on your hand without being afraid." Perhaps the butterfly needs less impeccable harmony than a bird for it to stay in place on a moving human being. Nevertheless, it can be assumed that in terms of the smooth shifting of my weight from one intricate form to another, and most importantly because of the controlled stillness of my torso and shoulders, the yin and yang were harmonious enough to make the butterfly not afraid.

The even breathing process is so intimately related to the action, at all times, that even the sensitive butterfly was unaware of it, and what sent it on its separate way was the sudden change of pace.

Such an experience illustrates the intrinsic nature of T'ai-Chi Ch'uan movement—that it succeeds in giving one the power to remain quiet and fluidly continuous whatever the yin-yang dynamic variations are and no matter how the pattern relationships change. And it is to be especially noted that quick motions in T'ai-Chi Ch'uan do not change the breathing rhythm and that what startled the butterfly was the unexpected *action*. *Nothing* in T'ai-Chi Ch'uan disturbs the natural heartbeat or the breathing tempo. This is due not only to the special timing of movement to movement and space to space but also to the fact that all is done without emotional content.

The ability to balance the interweaving action smoothly, to look as if all were executed with equal lack of intensity, is indeed part of the movement miracle. Actually the dynamic variations even in a small area are always moving from "empty" (slightly weighted) to "solid" (strongly grounded) as well as from lightness to power—all done according to physiological requirements and gravity's demands. The structured movements of T'ai-Chi Ch'uan regulate the opposites so that all become harmonious. It will always feel miraculous that the perpetual interaction of space-dynamics can be so impeccably controlled.

The movement is a miracle of function in respect to the physiological clarity with which the complex Forms can be executed. One is in constant wonder that even the most minute and delicate of Transitions, seemingly unseen, possess such "tangibility," the subtlety of which is both the cause and result of awakening awareness and deepening perception.

It is a moving miracle when T'ai-Chi Ch'uan structures can be applied so meticulously to our physiological and psychological selves that body stamina and mental ease are simultaneously developed.

The flow of movement is a miracle of balance—every unit of Form, every Transition being spatially and dynamically adjusted with mathematical exactitude to prevent the force of gravity from throwing one off one's "center," physically and mentally.

The way of T'ai-Chi Ch'uan is the essence of grace. Being smooth, even, light, and flowing would, it seems, be enough for a technique to be termed graceful, but the grace in T'ai-Chi Ch'uan evolves from the complex intricacies both of the Way and the movements which weave their curvilinear paths in inevitable harmony with space and time—a universal grace.

This essential grace, and with it dignity, permeates the self when the mind is present (as it must be) with the action.

The atmosphere created from mind-body grace is as restful and
secure as is the calm curve of the horizon and as contained as
the arc of the sky.

No less a miracle is the fact that the total personality is
always engaged with the process of the moving activity. No matter
what the technical concerns are, no matter where the emphasis
lies, and no matter how the mind moves, the self sustains a
feeling of wholeness. Even the merest beginner in this complex
art experiences at moments this intrinsic wholeness and is led by
such awareness to stay with the "long journey" and move toward
more profound and long-lasting perceptions.

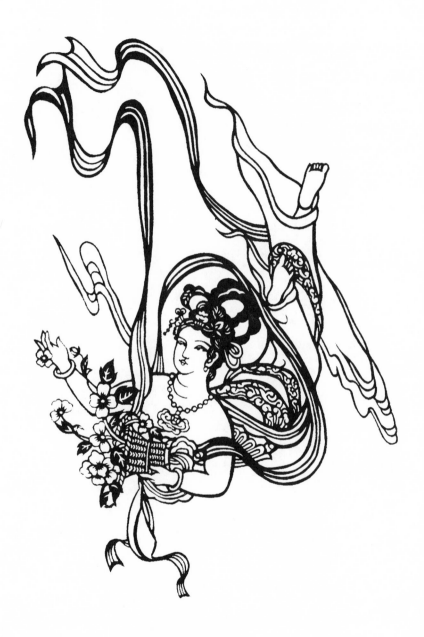

Timeless Ease

2. The Constant Curve: The Circle and the Wave

The design for the T'ai-Chi Ch'uan diagram is the subtle symbol for the balanced philosophy and the physiological processes which comprise T'ai-Chi Ch'uan. The double wave line centered in a circle epitomizes the grace of flowing space in all the structured action of this exercise-art. The boundary of the circle keeps shape and movement under control within its wholeness. The double turn within it makes a unity of forms move as if in unlimited and free exchange.

The circle and the wave produce all shades of differentiation in yin-yang interchange. Necessarily related, the dual activity of this dynamic interplay results in balance impeccably adjusted in the ever-changing patterns of this many-faceted composition.

The essence of unity is embodied in the concept of such duality—action-movement and the dynamic changes as wave, and stillness-quiescence as circle.

We weave a circle of containment around us as we follow the continuous circular paths which form T'ai-Chi Ch'uan structure. Unwittingly, we create a field of energy within us as we experience the rhythmic ebb and flow of the dynamic changes inherent in the nature of the wave.

When we perform with physiological accuracy the motion of wave and circle in their proper proportions, we will be in perfect coordinated balance. The circle is an urge to wholeness, and the wave is ceaseless change. The circle, though it may be thought of as a finite circumference, is yet capable of limitless expansion. The wave may seem boundless, but framed as it is by the embracing circle, it does have its spatial limitations.

The interweaving wave patterns have a destination—that of becoming Form. Form is the union of balanced space-time relationships that have momentarily culminated (climaxed) in a completed structure which is felt as total stillness (yin); the yang or motion patterns having gradually transformed themselves into yin structure. Form as an ending, however, does not cease or stop; its completeness, sensed, sets a new beginning into motion. It is as if one had rounded out a circle which, as Form, contains the seed of new action.

Form can be considered to express the contained and calm spirit of circle and motion, the process which materializes the form. The way of the wave action (which is what the T'ai Chi is) is the means by which to advance to the meaning. This is the heart of the process of T'ai-Chi Ch'uan.

The Forms (108 in all) are each a unique state of awareness. Each represents a peak experience in the evolving process of self-development which, like the circle, has unbounded possibilities for profound expansion.

"The T'ai-chi is the symbol of the universe"—Professor Joseph Needham

3. The Historically Accurate T'ai-Chi Circle

The symbol for the T'ai-Chi is a circle divided into curved shapes of equal size, one being yin, the shadowed right part, and the other yang, the light part. A touch of yin in yang and of yang in yin is indicated by the small dot of the opposite color in each area, showing the flexible and sympathetic character of each to the other. The line between them has the movement of a wave. The fall and rise of the wave line is also yin and yang; this flowing is restrained and contained by the evenness of the circumference. All of the movement represents the continuity of the life-force, which is *movement.*

Yin as the receptive, feminine, and yang as the creative, masculine, complement each other. Though opposite, they are not in opposition or antagonistic. Though different, they supplement each other in the continuous movement between them, without beginning and without end. When yang reaches its final moment, then yin is created and starts. The interplay of the two fundamental and vital elements implies "perpetual motion." Together in T'ai-Chi, where their relationship so perfect, they constitute equilibrium and harmony.

The symbol indicates that which is held in balance yet separated. A few examples of the opposite (placing yang before yin) as experienced in the exercise of T'ai-Chi Ch'uan are movement-stillness, motion-rest, tangible-intangible, straight-curved, expansion-contraction, inhilation-exhalation, outside-inside, solid-empty (void), light-dark, firm-soft, open-close, right-left, forward-backward, float-settle, and rise-sink. There is nothing without its opposite; nothing that does not change (move) in order to be permanent (to live)—which in itself is a yin-yang statement.

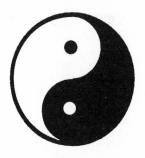

Fig. 4.1 The T'ai-Chi Symbol. The historically correct position for the T'ai-Chi symbol places the light portion (yang) rising up to heaven and the dark portion (yin) descending to earth.

In my long experience with teachers of T'ai-Chi Ch'uan in the United States, I have found few (if any!) who ever noticed the wave-curve, much less saw the way it was drawn. In recent years, some have taken for granted that it was an S curve, like the letter S in our alphabet. Very few have inquired into the history and philosophy of the T'ai-Chi symbol.

The current version of the T'ai-Chi symbol was designed during the Sung dynasty with the curve in a form similar to a reverse S. The symbol has so remained in all of classical Chinese literature. When books are translated into English, the printer usually makes the mistake of reversing the symbol. (How well I know printer's and publisher's errors, having experienced the horror of having many of my T'ai-Chi Ch'uan forms printed in reverse or backwards in my own publications, books and articles.)

In the book *T'ai-Chi Ch'uan, Its Effects and Practical Applications* (English edition, printed in Shanghai by Y. K. Chen) a short section on page five deals with the T'ai-Chi diagram:

> *There are two different Grand Terminus Diagrams in China. One, made in black and white circles, was designed by Chou Lien-ch'i, a notable scholar of the Sung Dynasty (A.D. 1017–1073). The other is the Double Fish*

Diagram adopted by the common folk. The former is
adopted by the Confucians, and the latter by the Taoists.
Though they differ in form, they are exactly the same in
representing the theories of Yin and Yang.

The symbol of Chou Lien-ch'i represents two gua from
the *I-Ching*, or *Book of Changes*, interchanging cosmic forces.
These two forms, or trigrams, are Fire (trigram from I-Ching) on
the page left in the yang position, and Water on the right in the
yin position. Fire and Water create steam, the symbolic repre-
sentation of unseen life-force as depicted in the ideograph for
the word qi.

The double fish diagram's upper curve with a reversed S
configuration is consistent with the art of Chinese calligraphy.
The dark side (yin) pertains to the left side of our bodies; the
light side (yang) to the right side.

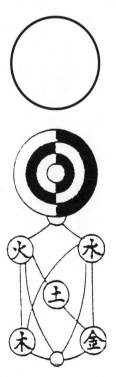

**Fig. 4.2 The Sung Dynasty Diagram
Depicting Yin/Yang, by Chou Lien-ch'i.
This symbol, adopted by most Confucians, represents the yang *gua*, Fire,
on the right with the yin *gua*, Water,
on the left.**

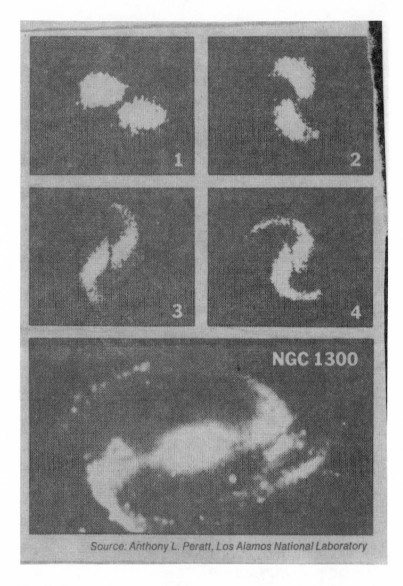

Fig. 4.3 This computer simulation shows how electromagnetic plasma forces interact to form a classical spiral galaxy. This is an actual model of the formation of Galaxy NGC1300. (*New York Times*, 28 February 1987). Copyright © 1987 by the New York Times Company. Reprinted by permission.

One very interesting note from the science of astrophys-
ics involved the creation of spiral galaxies. Computer simulations used in the study of the formation of spiral galaxies suggest
that the formation of these galaxies comes about through the
electromagnetic attraction of a charged gas or plasma which
creates a magnetic field. This highly charged energy field bends
plasma, forcing the entire mass to begin a spiral rotation. The
electronic simulations bear a startling resemblance to the formation of a double fish T'ai-Chi diagram in the classical yang right–
yin left configuration. Perhaps the universe knows something
about the Tao.

4. The Landscape of the Self in Spirit

This is a landscape of the self from the point of view of the state of mind in harmony with the designed-body action.

The duality of body and mind is made to balance with and through a vast number of differentiated concepts both structural and mental; each concept separately capable intrinsically of relating to any of the others. For example, we can speak of the curvilinear aspect of movement in T'ai-Chi Ch'uan structure and refer to "curve" as being peaceful, producing calmness. At the same time, we can also say that moving with consciousness of the curving connections will prevent and/or eliminate superfluous expenditure of energy. The curve aspect, therefore, is both emotional (mental) and physical (structural).

The landscape of the self I have devised is a "game of changing unities" to stimulate appreciation as to how compatible, meaningful, congenial the various concepts are—concrete-abstract, tangible-intangible—and how they can be juxtaposed, interchanged, and combined and how they contain and maintain intrinsic sense in their interchanges. They can be seen to relate in several ways—symbolically, literally, structurally, physically, and on emotional-mental levels.

Visualize "mind" as the hub of a wheel from which radiate the mental concepts which signify attention, awareness, patience, calmness, perception, alertness, equilibrium, clarity, concentration, tranquility, ease, and containment.

Visualize another wheel with "body" as the hub from which radiate: pattern-shape-form, space-direction, tempo, yin-yang dynamics, coordination, continuity-flow, curvilinear movement, balance, stillness, activity, diversity, and unity.

I have not, as you can see, used the "Wheel" to illustrate the concepts. I have instead (easier to handle) used a table: there are two rectangles, each divided into twelve parts; one rectangle is *Mind;* the other is *Body.* See table 4.1 and copy the chart on a separate sheet of paper and each item can then be used to focus on the instructions easily.

To play this Game of Changing Unities:

1. Cut out each item.

2. Put "Mind" in one envelope.

3. Put "Body" in another one.

4. The idea is to "blindly" take out one slip from each envelope and pair them. Note their relationship. For instance, *perception* may come out of envelope 1 and *tempo* out of envelope 2. Obviously, perception must be present to maintain tempo correctly, and perception is made keener by being able to maintain one tempo.

You can (1) keep one concept (either body or mind) and pair it with several from the other envelope any number of times, or (2) continue to pair all of them, one after the other, or (3) return the chosen slip to its envelope and start anew after shaking the envelope.

New insights will be awakened from this "game" as to the complex, organic relationships of all the qualities in T'ai-Chi Ch'uan—which, in one way or another, reveal the possibility of unending harmony of mind and body—on many intricate levels.

It is important to delve into the *spirit* of the interchanging relationships—to think, perceive, and, if one really knows T'ai-Chi Ch'uan *well* enough, experience the multiplicity that becomes a unity.

Table 4.1 The Game of Changing Unities 93

Mind

M Attention	M Awareness	M Patience
M Calmness	M Perception	M Alertness
M Equilibrium	M Clarity	M Concentration
M Tranquility	M Ease	M Containment

Body

B Pattern-Shape-Form	B Space-Direction	B Tempo
B Yin-Yang Dynamics	B Coordination	B Continuity-Flow
B Curvilinear Movement	B Balance	B Stillness
B Activity	B Diversity	B Unity

5. Finding the Straight in the Curved

I venture to give my thoughts and interpretation of finding the straight (path) in the curved (path)—but only from the point of view of the space-movement in T'ai-Chi Ch'uan's structure.

We know that any segment of this exercise can be treated analytically from other concepts—philosophical, physical, symbolic, and so on—all of which would contribute to the unity of the whole.

I shall, however, treat this subject only with the idea of the structured "plane" in which the particular part of the body moves. To be brief, I shall confine myself to the action of the arms and hands, as they function to create a Form.

The two *paths* of movement are the transitions destined to culminate in a complete wholeness of "Circle and the Wave," the T'ai-Chi position. (Fig. 4.4).

To make the matter clear as to the words *straight* and *straightened*: the full-length position of an arm, for instance, will be termed a straightened arm. The *path* the arm is made to take is designated as "straight."

To emphasize this, the term I am using is the path of action that a wrist and hand make as they traverse in space from one position to another. The *direction* of the circular or straight path may be horizontal, diagonal, or vertical.

Example:

1. Raise right straightened arm sideways—shoulder high—full length, with wrist straight and palm facing floor.

2. Bring wrist in toward shoulder, by bending elbow downward and bending wrist so that palm remains facing the floor. Move the arm inward close to body, so that elbow is close to side of torso, therefore wrist, too, will be as close to body as person's arm permits.

    Result: The hand and wrist have moved in a perfectly straight path from out to inward, horizontally, determined by wrist action. Note that the arm joints have been activated in proper sequence, that is, a wave action.

3. Reverse the action outward: Move finger tips outward by stretching elbow joint thus straightening wrist as well.

    Note:

    A. The hand itself can take other positions such as bending the wrist so that the hand is flexed with palm facing outward; or, turning palm upward or sideways with a straightened wrist.

    B. The path inward or outward is a straight one. It is the wrist (not the palm) which determines the path of activity inward; the fingers point outward.

The Curved Path of Movement

Example:

1. Extend the right arm outward, shoulder high, at full length with palm sideways facing forward and wrist straightened.

2. Bend elbow slightly so that the arm and hand are induced to move toward the *front*, at shoulder level; the arm begins to form an arc at the elbow joint.

3. Move the hand forward and in toward the left shoulder side so that the elbow becomes more of a curve; stop

movement when the elbow joint is slightly greater than a 90-degree angle. The arm now is in a full curve. (When elbow is at a 90-degree angle, it forms a right angle, i.e., squared.)

4. The path the arm has made, horizontally, is a curved path enfolding the torso.

5. A controlled curved arm when raised head high (from 4 above) would be moving in a curved path, vertically.

In other words, the curving path begins when we move the straightened arm into a curved form; and the completed curved form, when moved, also traces a curvilinear path—in any direction, up, sideways, downwards.

The straightened, fully positioned arm is said to move with "wavelike" action because wrist and elbow must be activated in order to be able to move in a straight path as described above: inward, outward, or downward.

Note these opposites:

1. The curved arm can hold its form when moving in a curved space.

2. The straightened arm must by itself, move the joints in wavelike action, to create a straight path.

We therefore, have relative stillness appearing in the curved action. We have yin-yang activity when the straight path is described. There is always a balanced harmony of the opposites in creating form and structure.

The following illustrations of "Finding the Straight in the Curved" are all from the Wu style of T'ai-Chi Ch'uan.

Experiencing the Straight Path as It Moves *into* the Curved Path

The right arm is a "wave" arm. The palm is turned outward with a bent wrist (yang), about 5–6 inches away from chest, at the heart (i.e., armpit) level. The elbow, therefore, is bent and is in the plane of the side of body.

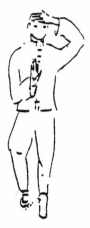

Fig. 4.4 The T'ai-Chi Form. The left arm is a curved arm, with a straightened wrist (yin) and palm facing the forehead; elbow points out diagonally forward; the hand is held a few inches away from the forehead.

Note that the right fingertips point upwards toward the left hand. They are in the same vertical plane. This form exemplifies the Circle and the Wave, that is the T'ai-Chi Form (Fig. 4.4.)

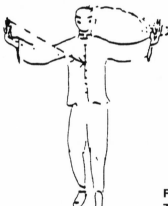

Fig. 4.5 How We Arrive at the T'ai-Chi Form (above)

Both arms move simultaneously, moving in a straight path with the right arm and in a curved path with the left arm.

1. *Position of arms:* Both arms are outstretched shoulder high, diagonally forward (northeast and northwest).

Palms (yang) face outward with bent wrists. (Note: I am not including leg action.) (Fig. 4.5.)

2a. *Movement of left arm:* Turn left palm to face inward while hand moves toward the forehead.

Bending left elbow slightly, bring hand with straightened wrist to forehead as in the curvilinear path described in Figure 4.5.

The elbow has been curving to become an obtuse angle. The path of the movement of the left hand goes from shoulder height to forehead level—in a curved path, diagonally upward.

2b. *Movement of the right arm:* Bend elbow downward and inward toward the torso, all the while moving the hand with palm out, in an inward straight path (diagonally). The hand travels to the chest, heart-level area, as described in Figure 4.4.

Here we have a straight path moving slightly diagonally downward and inward. The hand and wrist maintaining the straight path while the elbow becomes more fully bent. The elbow ends its position at the side of the torso. Right arm is a "wave."

The T'ai-Chi Form has been created by means of the passing of movements, in the curved and the straight paths, simultaneously. This is "Seeking the straight in the curved" and actually finding them when one understands the subtleties! The straight path has moved within the curve.

The Enfolding Form

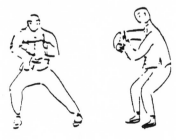

Fig. 4.6 The Enfolding Form (Completed Movement)

1. The torso is slightly bent forward from the waist (45-degree angle).

2. The right arm is circularly held at chest level with arm parallel to the floor; the right elbow is in the plane of the right shoulder, slightly lower. The right hand has a straightened wrist with palm facing inward toward the left side of body. Since this is a circular form, the right hand is farther out from the left shoulder than is the right elbow from the right shoulder. The elbow, therefore, is at an obtuse angle, that is, curved.

3. The left arm is "within" this arc of circle, the left palm faces the inner right elbow close to it. The left wrist is bent. The left elbow is bent downward at left side. Here we again have the right arm in a circle and the left arm in a wave. (Fig. 4.6.)

How We Arrive at the Enfolding Form

1. Start out from a position with arms slightly diagonally forward shoulder high with both hands turned upward with straight wrists. As torso bends forward, the arms will move simultaneously. (Fig. 4.7, the transition to Fig. 4.6, p. 99.)

2a. *The right arm:* Turn palm forward and curve arm as described in example 2 above, by bending elbow slightly and gradually curving arm to become a greater arc. This

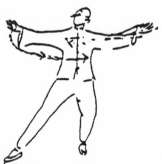

Fig. 4.7 How we arrive at the Enfolding Form

movement is exactly like the one described in example
2, except that here the torso will bend forward. The
curved arm is made to move in a curved path.

2b. *The left arm:* Bend left elbow downward, flexing wrist so
that palm faces and remains upward; wrist and hand lead
movement inward. Palm turns toward where the right
elbow is and will land; the arm, as a wave arm, is moved
by the palm. Wrist is moving in a straight path toward
the right-elbow position (from west to east).

Here we have a straight path moving horizontally into the
embrace of a curved arm on a curved path, culminating in a form
comprised of a circle and a wave, placed horizontally. This is in
contrast to the T'ai-Chi form (Fig. 4.4), which is on a vertical plane.

Transition to Fan Behind the Neck Form

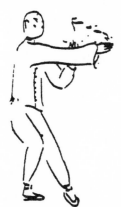

**Fig. 4.8 Transition to Fan Behind the
Neck Form**

1. Face diagonally left; or for the purpose of this exercise,
   one can face front. (This position follows the Golden
   Needle at the Bottom of the Deep Sea Form).

2. Place straightened right arm forward, shoulder high; palm
   faces sideways; wrist is straightened.

3. Place left palm at crook of right elbow; fingers point
   upward and wrist is flexed. Left elbow is bent and remains
   at left side, lower than level of wrist.

The Action of the Straight Path and the Curved Path
Simultaneously

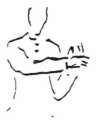

Fig. 4.9 The Simultaneous Action of the Straight Path (*on left*) and the Curved Path (*on right*) (also as in Fig. 5.19)

1a. Move right hand inward toward the left side of torso; palm faces inward toward torso—wrist remains straightened. Stop hand when it reaches a point which makes right elbow form a right angle (90-degrees). Hand will be level with elbow, therefore lower arm will be parallel to torso, at shoulder level. The hand has described an arc (inevitably), horizontally.

1b. The left hand, with palm facing outward, moves to left torso side, remaining at the same distance from the torso, because the hand moves in the plane of the right elbow; it is moving in a straight path from right to left side. The left elbow is down at the left side; the back of the hand faces the left shoulder.

Therefore, the palms face each other in a "cross," the right hand is horizontal, while the left hand is vertical. Both hands are at shoulder level.

The right hand described a curve while the left was moving in a straight path. The result is a straight path within the path of an arced circle.

I have limited my analysis of "straight and curved" paths to only three examples from which one can see how space-action-variety "works" in T'ai-Chi Ch'uan.

Throughout the structure, there are continually changing combinations as well, differently joined circle with circle (paths), straight with straight (paths) as well as the straight and curved: each is formed with diverse proportions of tempo, space-shape-size, yin-yang dynamics.

The entire composition, it must be remembered, is dominated by the curvilinear process—the "property" of the universe. And it is this process which creates calmness, containment, patience, and power.

It is the curvilinear—the arc, the wave, the parabola, ellipse, and so on—which are the means by which energy is *not* wasted but instead is built up, reserved, and stored.

The straight is a linear motion by which power is expended and externalized. The curve is containment, and limits the excessive force of the straight path by "embracing" it, that is, finding the straight in the curve.

T'ai-Chi Ch'uan can be performed agreeably without the player having any knowledge, awareness, or appreciation of the inner workings of the exercise.

We can look at a clock and know the time without knowing anything about its inner mechanism. We are "outside" of the clock's time-work.

However, obviously, since we are to become what T'ai-Chi Ch'uan promises and to participate in what is inherent in it, we must try to begin to inquire into what makes T'ai-Chi Ch'uan "tick" and we should be curious as to what lies beneath the surface of the "agreeable" feeling in order eventually to "possess" its qualities.

We must delve into the means and method by which the harmony of action and purpose has been created.

To look into a painting and comprehend its compositional organization, its color juxtaposition, or the subtlety of nuance, is to experience some deeper feeling than would have come from simply accepting the surface content (abstract or concrete).

The art of knowing enhances physical proficiency, emotional pleasure, and in due time will elevate the spirit.

The analytical studies of the various features of T'ai-Chi Ch'uan's structure and spirit will not interrupt the continuity of one's feeling, nor will it inhibit the ch'uan's (the action's) "spirit."

Knowledge of the way of the T'ai-Chi will enlighten us as to the harmonious interaction of the many layers of the activity: mental, physical, aesthetic, philosophical.

Such "knowingness" will gradually seep into the system and become one with the action, thus inevitably increasing the player's pleasure as well as competence. Such knowledge will develop a sensitivity in which higher levels of "comprehension" take root.

6. Form and Transition: Dual Themes in T'ai-Chi Ch'uan Structure

What is so specifically significant about the nature of the Form in T'ai-Chi Ch'uan that it is designated as such? Even new students feel "something" different from what they had been doing when they arrive at the position we call a *Form*. They simply stop moving, as if they had reached a destination. It is as if something had completed itself, producing in them a feeling of accomplishment and a sense of satisfaction.

That, and very much more, is what a Form "offers," as the player progresses to a stage of appreciating the cooperative relationship of Form and Transition.

The classic T'ai-Chi Ch'uan styles of Yang, Wu, Sun, and Ho comprise 108 Forms and an equal number of Transitions which follow each other in perfect alternating sequence.

Each Transition leads to the creation of a Form, which, in turn, sows the "seed" of the next Transition. The flowing complex formation of Transition gives rise to yet another Form— all throughout the exercise—from the very beginning of T'ai-Chi Ch'uan when a Transition (the first) moves from the basic position to create the first Form, named T'ai-Chi. At the conclusion of the exercise, the 108th Transition culminates in the 108th Ending Form (Complete Stillness).

Whereas the Transition is always in constant motion, the Form is "stillness" personified. It becomes stabilized in a "moment of time." Transitions move in space-time formations with varying degrees of dynamic yin-yang energy changes, and always with challenging complexities.

Form is distinguished by the simultaneous union of all elements within it: space-shape-pattern, dynamic variations so proportionately balanced as to seem to erase the individuality of each element, blending all into "oneness" and so causing the form to be "stilled."

This suspended action is intrinsic to all Forms. Although the physical configurations are different in each, the awareness produced within each is similarly felt. Each structured Form develops individually from the process—the Transition—which precedes it all through the exercise as has been noted, each progressing in an evolutionary way.

Just as the physical self becomes more stable and more secure during the long exercise with its diversity of movements, so the mind and spirit become more centered, sensitized, and alert (subtle and illuminated), as T'ai-Chi Ch'uan progresses to become a "higher" experience.

Form, in contrast to the yang of Transition, is of the yin element—the entity of quietness and repose. The interrelated aspects which comprise the Form are fused, unified at a simultaneous movement. The Form feels so "finished" that the player is momentarily held at a "stand-still" (never apparent to a viewer).

Although the essence of Form and Transition differ as to substance and spirit, they nevertheless are integrated themes in keeping with the philosophy of the "balance of the opposites," through the interplay of yin-yang elements and the intrinsic nature of the compositional choreography as required by the harmony of the whole.

It may not be too farfetched to say that they—Form and Transition—represent in tangible form the Circle and the Wave, as delineated in the diagram which symbolically illustrates the concept of T'ai-Chi, the philosophy of the intrinsic (universal) balance of activity and stillness in harmony. The diagram is a *circle* embracing a wave, the action of which is perpetual within the still completeness of the circle.

Form is the yin of the circle which expresses (and is) self-containment, completeness. Transition is the yang of the wave, the ever-moving path: the constant interchange of all phenomena.

T'ai-Chi Ch'uan epitomizes the way and the content of the philosophy of the T'ai Chi, and that is why T'ai-Chi Ch'uan—this Ch'uan—is different from all the hundreds of other Ch'uan (exercises) in China. This Ch'uan designated as T'ai Chi is the only Ch'uan of its kind.

Forms are the 108 "stations" in and on the path of the continually active Transitions. Together, both the moving path and the station, which is the destination, express the meaning of substance and spirit, the purpose and the goal, the means and the end of T'ai-Chi Ch'uan, to which the mind-heart-body behavior is directed.

The intrinsic stillness of the "station," as Form, complements the flowing path of transition, the ever-interweaving chain of action. If one were to "stop" this movement at any point of its journey, the arrested attitude would feel artificially stilled, unfinished as a position, urging the body to "go" ahead— somewhere.

A Form held beyond its time will never stir any mental need for moving out of it. Some of the elements which compose the Form are in impeccable "union." The position has, so to speak, no "future to come," as the Transition has, prodded by unresolved physicality. The Form is self-sufficient, "emptied" of all differences, awakening feelings of peacefulness, calmness, a sense of equilibrium.

To explain the "balance of stillness" as is experienced in a Form, I suggest the "physical" image of a horizontal scale at each end of which rests an object—one being large like a pound of feathers, the other being small, like a pound of iron. Note that the objects, different as to bulk or quality, are of *equal* weight. The scale is absolutely still—as if nothing were on it. The different features of a Form, legs in different altitudes or shaped at different levels, and hands and wrists at different angles; all, together, are *gravitationally* weighted, equally. The significance of the Form in each of the 108 is that of "weight-lessness." The player experiences a Form position as the nonaction of a balanced scale—quiet, ease, and restfulness. With develop-ing knowledge, awareness, and sensitivity, one moves inexorably, with the substance of action toward the spirit of containment—heart and mind ease emptied of "negative" emotions.

The names of the Forms as popularly given are symbolic handles by means of which one is apprised of the presence of a Form. The essence of the meaning of the Form will gradually be awakened by experience and the symbolic names will be more than guideposts.

The names as given "publicly," metaphors, symbols, po-etic allusions to their true meanings, are never revealed to a young student. Why is this so?

If the student were to know beforehand what to expect at various times, and how to experience (or put to use) certain emotional and mental states, it stands to reason that a conscious question, a certain goal, would deceive the player into thinking that he/she had had a "true experience."

The act of doing T'ai-Chi Ch'uan gives knowledge to one's self, as awareness of what is being achieved in mind and body develops. The all-pervading structure on numerous levels will by itself awaken the promised qualities of the known goals, which appear even in the least astute beginner. A few of these are:

Patience—through the coordination aspect;

Attention—through the variety of patterns, positions and Forms;

Endurance—through the time-length of the exercise;

Stamina—through the complexities of body movements;

Ease and quiet—as described in Forms;

Perseverance and will-power—built up gradually.

All develop *without* intellectual striving. Understanding and knowledge develop organically because of the innate har-mony of every aspect of action in T'ai-Chi Ch'uan.

In the composite architecture of the composition, the content of Transition and Form has even further significance, more than what is separately portrayed.

Transition, the yang element, "uses" in the interweaving process *both* small yin and yang changes, which produces a flowing energy in the motion. Form, totally yin, has erased all dualities of "expression" within the Form structure itself. Its spirit is yin.

Since calmness, stillness, mindfulness suffuse the spirit of the Form, we can dare to call it "heavenly." This quality, however, cannot exist without another "opposite" process taking place, the presence of the "earthly." Transition exemplifies this—the body of action, thought, stamina is indeed "earthly." There is no state of pure independence of any aspect described since one element depends on some other, large or small, heavenly universal or earthly, in the dual themes: Form-Transition, Substance-Spirit, Action-Stillness. Each exists because of the other. All act in harmony within the philosophy of T'ai-Chi Ch'uan.

The following paragraph sums up (in part) the distinguishing characteristics of Form (yin) and Transition (yang)—listed in that order. To do so is not to separate them, but to clarify the nature of their relationship in the structure as a whole, so as to enrich the player's perception of "multiplicity in unity." The dual themes function organically with balanced consistency:

Spirit and substance; stillness and activity; state of being and state of becoming; quality of void/emptiness (Hsu) and the quality of weightedness (gravity); quiet mind and alerted mind; simplicity and intricacy; completion and process; effect (result) and cause; energy stabilized and energy created; feeling of permanence and feeling of transience; time arrested and time flowing; no distinction of "opposites" and definite division of opposites; feeling presence of "inner" self and feeling presence of one's physical body; destination (the station) and the moving pathway of "travel"; the containment or permanence of a "circle" and the ever-moving path of a wave (united in T'ai-Chi).

T'ai-Chi Ch'uan is a synthesis of opposites and of similarities as well. The most important example of this is the nature of all movement, "flowing like a gentle stream" in every formation.

The motion of muscular tension (great or small) is termed *intrinsic*, that is, made/changed naturally according to the requirements of the particular "bit" of action, not more, not less, at the moment.

Both still Form and moving Transition "use" the natural progress of dynamics in common: tension is never superimposed (extrinsically), never *forced* at any time unless dictated by the Form structure itself, which occurs exactly nine times (the creative exceptions).

Knowing, being aware of how the complex structure is "built," will surely help the conscientious player experience his/her function. Knowing augments the experience which moves toward attaining profound comprehension of more than the physical. And, to put it lightly, will prevent the exercise from ever becoming boring or automatic!

Structured Harmony

CHAPTER V

THE ORGANIC FLOW OF PHYSIOLOGY

Lightly, evenly, and in balance,
With liquid continuity, patterns
Pass from one part of the body
To the other, each growing out of
That which went before. The subtle
Sequence of this chain unfolds
Invisibly as does the change
From day to dusk to dark to light,
Smooth as a ring of cloudless sky
     The atmosphere of peaceful quiet
     Pervades the Being and the Movement
     At each measured moment—
     The right gesture
     At the right time
     In the right place
     For the right reason, all together
     Simultaneous and synchronized
          Is the art of grace refined.

The Organic Flow of Physiology

1. How Slow Is Slow?

T'ai-Chi Ch'uan is a slow, intrinsic exercise as distinguished from fast, extrinsic exercising. There is no difficulty in perceiving how fast a fast exercise is or in understanding the tensed nature of extrinsic action. The slowness and the variations of slow in T'ai-Chi Ch'uan are more difficult to apprehend and experience since it requires awareness of the muscle-release of superfluous tenseness as well as the control of a basic "nonquickness," both of which permit the movement to move continuously.

Most people are accustomed to expend themselves needlessly and are numb to their excessive tensions. The very first aspect to be considered in T'ai-Chi Ch'uan is its *basic* tempo, which can be acquired by those who are accustomed to move quickly (either through nervousness or temperament) and by those who are overly slow through lack of coordination. Both types can adapt themselves to the necessary basic tempo for many reasons, one of which is that it arouses a feeling of agreeable ease.

How slow is slow for beginners, advanced students, or experts, is a varying and developing matter. T'ai-Chi Ch'uan's *basic* tempo is based on the rapport between the fundamental tempo of the "inner" body and the outside movement so that at no point during the entire exercise are the heart and breath stirred up beyond their natural rhythms.

How slow is this slowness? It will take 22 to 25 minutes to perform the 108 Forms (no matter which school or style), depending on the extent of the subtleties included. At this tempo, no gesture combination will disturb the normal breathing time. This tempo can easily be taught from the very first movement by the "conscious" teacher.

To sustain it is a matter of awareness, attention, and prowess. A beginning student who tries to move too slowly will become overtense and will perspire profusely, which is always a sign of over-working. Only as one masters the exercise and oneself physically and psychically should one slow down and that should be done gradually over long practice, minute by minute.

Naturally, the physical aspect is being continually developed in terms of muscle-joint flexibility and strength. Also, with the basic tempo comes a perfect time-sense. Similarly, the mental concept of the structure in space and time, with yin-yang values in equilibrium, is simultaneously progressing. Without such knowledge and experience, T'ai-Chi Ch'uan can become, if the student works too slowly, a "mess" of tempo because then the Forms and patterns easily deteriorate into generalized designs without subtlety.

The gradual warming up of the body and the slow release of perspiration are two of the great advantages of this exercise where all is done at the right time and nothing is excessive—dynamics and pace being in harmony with the form.

As one becomes more expert, physically and mentally, only then should the tempo be slowed down ... by five minutes ... ten ... and so on, and this must be gradual as one masters the self. Before its time, very slow movement can be damaging since it requires a special kind of effort and concentration. The heart will tighten and the body will be exhausted if the whole being is not ready for it physically.

So, the beginner must be patient and calm enough to practice properly in basic tempo for inner harmony to be awakened. In doing T'ai-Chi Ch'uan in 25, 30, 40 or more minutes, one should feel as if one were moving on a "magic carpet" in space—light but secure, flowing but stable ... all in good tempo. This will be achieved all in "good time."

2. The Life of the Hand: Its Significance in T'ai-Chi Ch'uan

I have analyzed in detail the relationship of the hands to the general movements of T'ai-Chi Ch'uan in terms of the dynamics of change. Every hand form is as useful to the application of T'ai-Chi Ch'uan as an art of self-defense as it is to exercise for body-mind health.

Grandmaster Ma Yueh-Liang (Shanghai, China) in his recent book, *Wu Style—T'ai-Chi Ch'uan* (pp. 26–31), clearly defines the use of hands, their positions, and the nature of yin-yang qualities. Grandmaster Ma is a world-renowned master of T'ai-Chi Ch'uan in its defensive martial arts orientation. He is also well known as a superior master of Ch'i Kung.

Sensitivity to "how" the hands work is as important as the knowledge of how legs function for stability, defense, attack, balance, and security.

The knowledge of the intricacies in T'ai-Chi Ch'uan is not isolated from its practical use materialistically.

What was spontaneously said by a friend visiting me in Shanghai was one of my first encounters with the presence of T'ai Chi Ch'uan. Little did I understand the statement since I had just arrived and I had only seen T'ai-Chi Ch'uan mentioned in a guide book.

Apropos of some talk of my dance career and interest in the content and aesthetics of classical Chinese theater, Mei Ling animatedly said, "You should know the T'ai-Chi Ch'uan movement. When one moves in its form and method, properly and feelingly, one's inner energy can be projected outward through the very fingertips," and without much ado she then demonstrated several complex movements, marvelously slowly and flowingly, from which I could see both large forms and the subtle hand movement-changes.

I have learned through my many years of conscientious T'ai-Chi Ch'uan practice the significance and import of that inspired remark, which has remained in my "brain," to rise again and again when my experience was ripe enough to appreciate it.

The "hand" analysis that follows, however, is concerned with the practical "means" which will eventually lead to that above-mentioned perceptive aim. The physicality of hands in subtle movements functions as an integral part of a particular pattern with which they are involved structurally.

The greater the experience of the intricate way the different parts of the body behave in T'ai-Chi Ch'uan, the more profound will the player's responses be, physiologically, philosophically, psychologically, and aesthetically.

To be able to move "mentally" from the easy recognition of the obvious—the broad, open Forms—to the subtle and minute changes of movement relationships surely indicates the development of body sensitivity and mind astuteness. Awareness, in a practical way, of the integrated combinations of form in time and space with dynamics will determine the extent and the quality of one's well-being.

One of the many (subtle) concerns in rendering T'ai-Chi Ch'uan accurately, is how to make the hands function intelligently with conscious form, as an integrated element in the composite movement. For instance, in the Wu style of T'ai-Chi Ch'uan, hands are never permitted to relax gravitationally, like a loosened leaf hanging from a tree twig, nor are they considered merely adjuncts, as decorations attached to the arms. The hands in T'ai-Chi Ch'uan are never to be "emotional" as they are in "life"— capable of expressing fear, anxiety, nervousness, humility, anger,

love, sorrow, and so on. In T'ai-Chi Ch'uan, the hands have a
vital *function*—as vital as more compact parts of the body—vital
as the shoulders, waist, knees, all physiologically part of our structured beings. Knowledge of correct hand manipulation is as essential and important as obeying the physical methods of maneuvering
the legs, feet, torso, pelvis, head. The follow-through of hand
control to the very fingertips will perhaps be understood from the
following analysis of shape and dynamics of palm (the heart of the
hand), the dynamics and shape of the wrist, and the direction in
which the hand is made to move.

The physical variety of hand movements in the T'ai-Chi
Ch'uan system of which I am a longtime exponent—Wu (Chien-
Ch'uan) style—is basic to all styles. I shall deal with and explain
the way the hand-shapes, wrists, palms, and fingers change according to direction, form, dynamics of yin-yang. And how structure
and force of gravity determine the quality of the circulation of
yin-yang energy, which can penetrate through the very fingertips.

I suggest that since this is a "practical" essay, the reader
try to follow the explanation of the hand positions by doing
them physically, in order to appreciate their incipient power.
Suffice it to say that the T'ai-Chi Ch'uan student (or expert)
will come to recognize that the hands significantly contribute to
the awakening of awareness and calmness.

Analysis of Hand Forms

The cleverly organized hand forms have an intrinsic relationship
with the bodily patterns, positions, and configurations. It almost
goes without saying that every turn of the hand and wrist affects
the muscular activity of the entire arm, as well as the structure
of the whole.

Hands and wrists may be categorized: (1) as *having* yin or
yang energy, as well as neutral energy; (2) as *being* in a yin, or
yang, or neutral direction. The movement and position determine the energy "value"; the placement of the palms (the heart
of the hand) determines the nature of the yin or yang and neutral
direction.

1. Yang energy: The wrist is flexed so that the hand forms an angle to it. The palm may face outward, upward, downward, or inward.

2. Yin energy: The wrist is straight with its natural "softness" so that hand is in a direct line with the lower arm. The hand must not tip sideways.

3. Neutral energy: The wrist is straight as in yin energy, with hand in direct line with lower arm. The direction determines the "neutral."

Direction—As It Applies to the Palm

1. Yang direction for yang hand: The palm can face outward, away from body, or upward, inward (the wrist is flexed).

2. Yin direction for yin hand: The palm can face inward toward the body, or downward.

3. "Neutral" direction: The palm faces sideways, or at a diagonal.

Combination of Energy and Direction

1. Yang energy in a yang direction:

   (a) Wrist is flexed with palm facing outward; fingertips pointed upward.

   (b) Wrist is flexed with palm facing upward.

2. Yang energy in a yin direction.

   (a) Wrist is bent and palm faces downward.

   (b) Wrist is bent and palm faces inward.

3. Yin energy with yin direction.

   (a) Palm faces inward toward body, with a straight wrist.

   (b) Palm faces downward, with straight wrist.

4. Yin energy with yang direction.

   (*a*) Palm faces upward with straight wrist.

5. "Neutral" energy and neutral direction.

   (*a*) Wrist is straight, palm faces either sideways or on a diagonal.

6. Yang energy in a neutral direction.

   (*a*) Palm faces sideways; wrist is bent sideways. Fingers can point forward, diagonally downward, or diagonally upwards.

(*Note*: An aspect that affects the *degree* of energy used depends upon the force of gravity. Suffice it to say that when an arm is held vertically downward—no matter what the hand is doing—the energy exerted intrinsically is less than when an arm is horizontal or moving upward. Nevertheless, the *form* of the position is not changed.)

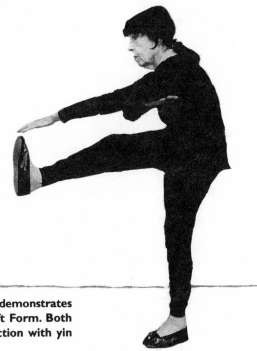

Fig. 5.1 Ms Delza demonstrates the Lotus Leg Lift Form. Both hands in yin direction with yin energy.

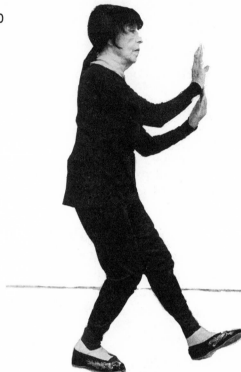

Fig. 5.2 Hand Strumming the Lute Form. Right hand in yang direction with yang energy; left hand in yin direction with yin energy.

The combinations of yin-yang variations in hand form and direction are sometimes subtle, as in transitions, and sometimes overt, as in Forms. They are as important to the dynamic body movement-positions (and the spirit of T'ai-Chi Ch'uan) as are the tempo regulation, the structural continuity, and the action of any single part of the body-action, one to the other—all of which make the whole a true harmony.

Explanation of the Palm and Hand Dynamic Relationship

The above-analyzed combinations of hand-wrist-energy-direction affect changes in the palm, aptly called the heart of the hand. This heart-palm is a significant area (perhaps one of the most important ones) which helps to maintain calm control and, by the subtle change in dynamics of movement, improves the circulatory processes.

1. Yang hand and yin palm: When the wrist is flexed and palm faces outward, upward, or downward. The palm has a quiet, full curve, with arced fingers *fulfilling the curves*, and "soft" knuckles. The yang hand energy is balanced by having a full yin palm.

2. Yin hand and "less" yin palm: When hand is yin—with straight wrist, the palm contains a shade of yang energy. The palm is *less curved* than in a yang palm, to balance the yin of wrist and yin direction. Palm therefore has a slightly "shallow" curve. There is, as a result, a balance in the dynamics of yin and yang.

3. Yin hand and yang direction (with palm more yin): When the arm (as an example) is outstretched sideways shoulder high, with straight wrist and palm facing upward. The palm, being in a yang direction, needs *less yang*, and is therefore more of a Yin palm.

4. The neutral or "standing" hand: The hand with its straight wrist has a less curved palm than does the yin hand. A more straightened palm is yang. The neutral hand always moves to become either a yang or a yin hand. The quality of the palm is changing continuously, going to, or from curved palm in a yang hand to, or from a less curved palm in a yin hand. The subtleties seem boundless in hand manipulations.

5. The grasping hand: This is a yang energy hand with a soft yin curved palm. The wrist is bent with fingers pointing downward, gathered together around the thumb-tip. The thumb touches the last two joints of the two inner fingers (the third and fourth). The thumb is straight; the knuckle of the other fingers are bent. The palm is hollow.

6. Hand positions, formed with tenseness:

   (*a*) When fingers are separated from each other, an added natural tenseness is required of the muscles and tendons. This kind of tension is an "intrinsic" matter—simply because fingers cannot be pulled apart unless they are activated with extra effort. The palm is straightened.

(b) Hands with fingers held together are consciously tensed in certain forms. Such intensity added to a gesture stiffens the palms and knuckles. This tension is termed "extrinsic."

7. The action of the fist-form:

(a) The fisted hand is held lightly, the bent-over fingers folding naturally over the palm. There is no added pressure. The heart-palm is yin and curved. The wrist is straight (usually). When hand is bent upward with fist-palm outward the hand is yang. The fist-palm may be faced upward or sideways.

(b) In Wu style, there are two strongly tensed fists which come with accented, speedy motion. The hand therefore is tensed to its fullest extent; the wrist is straight. The action is extrinsic.

The Natural T'ai-Chi Ch'uan Hand

All the variations of the hand-palm-wrist action flow from the position of the natural T'ai-Chi Ch'uan hand. Ordinarily when the arms hang vertically with palms turned toward the body, it is to be noted that the palms are curved with the fingers relaxed. But the T'ai-Chi Ch'uan hand is not like this "gravitationally relaxed" hand. Conscious effort is used to straighten the fingers slightly, which in turn lengthens the palm. The hand is now in a "neutral" position.

When the hands (palms) are turned to face rear, the hands will have a "life" (an energy) of their own: this is the T'ai-Chi Ch'uan hand, alert and ready for action.

Conclusion

The versatile hand is always at the service of the will and the mind. Its immediate response is ever present—"to give and take"

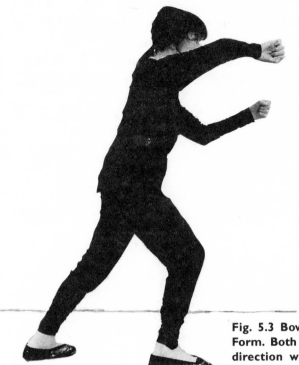

Fig. 5.3 Bow Shape Curve Form. Both feet in neutral direction with lesser yang energy.

in countless physical ways as well as to express emotions and ideas. Awareness of the cause for action is rarely recognized in everyday activity—as, for instance, reaching, grasping, clutching, and so forth, and at another level, stepping on or off a curb. Always mind-propelled, the body has been informed to act— with the speed of light.

In T'ai-Chi Ch'uan, the hand, also directed by mind, functions *impersonally*, as a part of the harmonious organization of bodily movements, intelligently integrated with the patterns, dynamics, tempo, and the "spirit" of T'ai-Chi Ch'uan; no emotional expressivity is ever projected into position or form.

The necessity to manipulate an immense variety of subtle gestures increases the depth of concentration and ease of complex coordination, both of which contribute to mental and emotional stability. Furthermore, keen perception of the essential relationship of the hand to the entire structure can, in due time, awaken a flow of a higher form of energy (perhaps magnetic) which ultimately can be projected "outward through the very fingertips."

As the Chinese say, "The hand is the extension of the will."

3. The Presence of the Eyes in the Action of T'ai-Chi Ch'uan

In taking the basic position at the start of T'ai-Chi Ch'uan, the stance, torso, spine-shoulder, hand and head positions should be given particular attention. So should the eyes. That we lose track of them during the action, especially in the early learning process, is readily "forgivable." The subtlety of the eye-muscle movement and the necessity of the mind's presence behind the eye-action need not be emphasized until that time when the T'ai-Chi Ch'uan player is prepared, physically and mentally, to experience many of the subtler aspects of the exercise: the smooth balance of the continuous motion, the physiological correctness of the forms, the space-tempo relationships, awareness of stillness in action, and the ability to function "intrinsically," that is, without false effort. An unmistakable *look* will itself develop when one feels the harmony of what is being done. The eyes will be alert, calm, knowing, and poised.

I have, in various essays, given thought to the various structural elements of T'ai-Chi Ch'uan from the point of view of physiology and philosophy. I have closely examined the subtleties in T'ai-Chi Ch'uan's weaving forms and patterns; I have pictured the ever-moving yin-yang elements in "The Life of the Hand." Now I venture to analyze more or less scientifically what happens in and to the eyes in a physical way during the active variations of movement.

Just as the physical body acquires a spirit in doing T'ai-Chi Ch'uan, so the eyes (or the mind's eye) become and remain alert, peaceful, and contained. The eyes can never be vacuous in T'ai-Chi Ch'uan, nor will they express anxiety or worry even while one is trying to remember and coordinate, though the eyes can, as we know, radiate any emotion: from hate to love plus all the emotions in between. The spirit of the movement in T'ai-Chi Ch'uan seeps through the whole physical being. Therefore, the eyes—regardless of the physical changes occurring—will feel light, secure, and impersonal. All of this is brought about naturally, not solely by emotional means, but through one's complete physical being.

The regulation of eye movements is as clearly organized in the structure of T'ai-Chi Ch'uan as is the play of every part of the body—large or small—contributing to physical and mental harmony.

The eyes seem to be so quietly set and unmoving during the activity that they are oftentimes outside of one's notice—both the performer's and the observer's. Should the eyes, however, shift randomly or dartingly, the overall impression would be one of nervousness, uncertainty, or restlessness.

Eye movements are unnoticed not because there is so much to do and/or observe in the ever-changing patterns of the exercise, but because they are focusing quietly and being instinctively controlled by the smooth consistency required of all T'ai-Chi Ch'uan movement changes.

The word "eyes," as used here, refers to all aspects of their physical composition—eyelids, eyeballs, and the muscles (which control the eye's ability to focus far or near, upward, downward, sideways or obliquely)—as well as emotions which can affect their appearance.

In the action of T'ai-Chi Ch'uan, all motion is intrinsically balanced, where form creates the continual variations of yin-yang dynamics, where extremes of tension are never required or permitted, and so it is with the use of the eyes, which respond intrinsically to the necessity of the movement at the moment.

Superfluous effort of any kind is not needed to regulate or stimulate the eyes, nor is it ever part of the action of the eyes, such as lowering the eye to look straight down at the body or raising the lids to see far upward at a 180-degree angle. Both movements are *extreme*.

The eye muscles are gently manipulated, always in basic slow tempo, adjusted to move or not to move with the body, responding to form, pattern, space, and direction, unless otherwise directed by the requirement of the particular position of the body and head. (This is explained later.) As indicated, the eyes behave in an organically instinctive and intrinsic way, in accord with the nature of T'ai-Chi Ch'uan, which is termed a "soft-intrinsic" system of activating the body for physical, emotional and mental well-being.

It is more difficult to experience the "soft-intrinsic" variation in the play of the eyes than it is, obviously, to feel the dynamic changes in the constantly manipulated body-forms. Just as physical action is not animated by an extrinsic force, so the eyes similarly maintain a calm, "impersonal" and therefore natural ease. When frowning, peering, straining, and otherwise expressing strong emotions do not disrupt intrinsic integrity and equilibrium, then the total being can achieve, through T'ai-Chi Ch'uan's harmonious principles, health and superior awareness.

The Basic Eye Position

The way the head is held at all times (with a few exceptions) affects the basic eye position. The head must be held erect, upright, so that the crown of the head is directed upward vertically as if attached by a "silken cord to the heavens." The chin, therefore, is not pressed inward toward the neck, nor is it tilted upward. The shoulders are low and relaxed, and the neck light. The mouth remains closed with the tip of the tongue lightly resting against the upper palate. With this perfect carriage of the head, the eyes will experience subtle muscular activity but outwardly will appear unchanged.

The overall eye position from which the dynamic variations occur is determined by the way the lids are held or moved. The gaze, in the basic eye position, is lowered to a 45-degree angle. (When the eyes are wide open and look directly forward, the gaze is at a 90-degree angle.) The eyes, with the gaze at a 45-degree angle, can see out at a long diagonal, downward path and come to rest on the ground approximately ten or twelve feet from where one is poised. The eye muscles will feel light and untaxed. They are in a "neutral" position.

The eyes maintain a gaze of 45-degrees 90 percent of the time during the exercise. We know that the ears hear without effort. So too, the eyes can see without any effort (Fig. 5.4.)

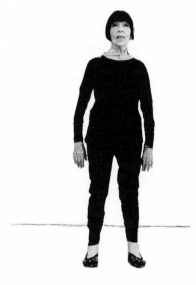

Fig 5.4 The Basic Eye Position as illustrated in the beginning form of T'ai-Chi Ch'uan.

Features of Eye-Behavior*

I. The Quiet Unmoving Eyes: When the eyelids, eyeballs, and eye muscles are not activated and the eyes are directed downward in the basic 45-degree seeing position.

    1. In a position where the body does not move out of place during a series of arm-leg movements, the eyes will be

---

*Note: All explanations and illustrations are based on the Wu system of T'ai-Chi Ch'uan

"fixed," looking downward at a 45-degree angle, focusing on an unspecific area on the ground. This is "pure" stillness of the quiet eye.

2. When the knees bend and the figure remains in the same space, the eyes do not change, but simply see a different area, slightly nearer than when the legs are straight. This, too, is "pure" stillness of the eyes. (Fig. 5.5.)

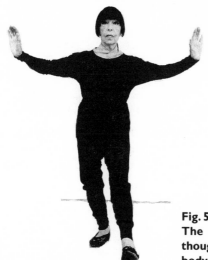

Fig. 5.5 Quiet, Unmoving Eyes. The eyes remain "still" even though the knees bend or the body turns.

3. When the entire figure turns, let us say, to the right side, if the body level remains the same, the eyes will simply see another area, without any eye-muscle movement. The gaze is quietly set and remains lowered 45 degrees during the movement.

4. When the movement is such that the entire figure moves forward or backward, as in *Brush-Knee-Twist (Walking-Step form)*, the eyes do not stir. One sees different areas on the ground farther forward as one advances, farther backward as one retreats. The path of vision remains still. (Fig. 5.6.)

The above illustrations emphasize the fact that the eyes and the unchanging muscles have remained still, quiet, and light. Such conscious control helps to create calmness.

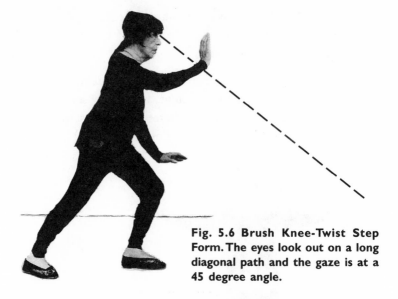

Fig. 5.6 Brush Knee-Twist Step Form. The eyes look out on a long diagonal path and the gaze is at a 45 degree angle.

II. The Quietly Moving Eyes: Muscles react with changes in body positions

1. In the Hand Strums the Lute Form, a hand moves into the basic line of vision, thus "forcing" an eye-muscle reaction. In figure 5.7, the player has taken a *Walking Stance*,

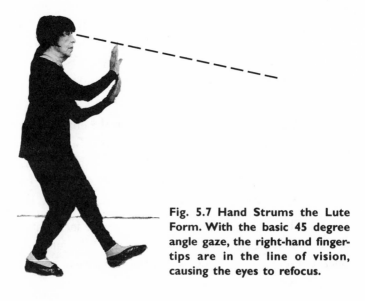

Fig. 5.7 Hand Strums the Lute Form. With the basic 45 degree angle gaze, the right-hand fingertips are in the line of vision, causing the eyes to refocus.

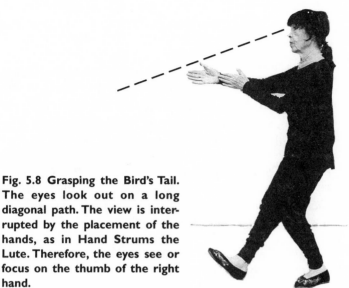

Fig. 5.8 Grasping the Bird's Tail. The eyes look out on a long diagonal path. The view is interrupted by the placement of the hands, as in Hand Strums the Lute. Therefore, the eyes see or focus on the thumb of the right hand.

with the right arm placed outward shoulder high. The eyes are free to gaze along the basic 45-degree path. The figure then sits back into an Empty Step form, at the same time bringing the right hand to center, in front of the nose and chin, blocking the line of vision. The eyes are then "forced" to see the tips of the fingers; this activates the eye-muscles. When the hand is removed, the eyes refocus. But "interference" in the line of vision automatically activates the muscles to become tense. (Fig. 5.7.)

2. The eye action in the Hands Strum the Lute form occurs frequently with variations, more or less tensed depending on the form. For example, in the Wu style's third series, when a leg is outstretched and an arm is extended shoulder high with the head turned toward it, the eyes have a "longer look" and are focused on the thumb of that hand; thus the tension in the eye muscles is lessened. The eye muscles are often stirred by a variety of movements. The eyes are less tense when looking at an object which is far away than when seeing one that is close. The eye muscles are never overworked

in T'ai-Chi Ch'uan since no positions are repeated successively.

3. When the torso sinks or bends forward or sideways and the head and neck remain still, the eyes will, then, see the ground closer to the feet, thus activating the eye muscles, as illustrated above in figures 5.4 and 5.5. The gaze will remain at a 45-degree angle.

In all the above illustrations, the *look* has remained unaltered—quiet and calm; the feeling of stillness predominates. All the action, light or strong, is intrinsic, that is, done according to the physiological laws of nature.

III. The Active (Willed) Eye Movements: The eyes are directed to bestir themselves in coordination with certain movements and forms.

1. The Wu Style Cloud-Arms Form. At certain times the eyes move from a 45-degree gaze to an open-eyed 90-degree gaze in the following way. The eyes look at the palm of the left hand, which is placed near the outstretched right arm. The left hand is then moved toward

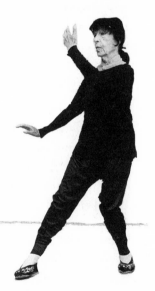

Fig. 5.9 Cloud Arms Form. The eyes see the palm of the left hand, which is held about twelve inches away from the face. The eyes are opened wide in a 90 degree gaze.

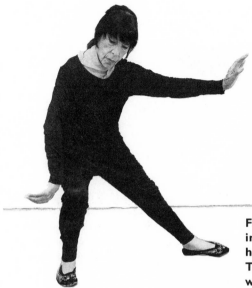

Fig. 5.10 Transition to Flying Oblique Form. The head is slightly tucked in. The eyes see the right wrist.

the face, the palm as high as the eyes and about ten to twelve inches away. This eye-level position raises the gaze to a 90-degree angle. Throughout this Form, the eye muscles are being activated both to "rest" by returning the eyes to the 45-degree gaze, and to be stirred to a 90-degree gaze, and finally to allow the eyes to look far into the distance, thus resting the eyes fully. Such changes, by being consciously directed, extend the range of eye exercise movements.

2. In the Flying Oblique Form, the body position is held unchanged as the right foot, right hand, and head are moved. The head is tipped downward slightly toward the right side. The eyes look down obliquely at the upturned right palm, which is in front of the right knee. Throughout this complex moving Form, the head and eyes hold their position in respect to the right hand, while the torso is regulated to release pressure in the neck. The Form ends with the eyes seeing the back of the right hand, the head still slightly tipped. The eyes

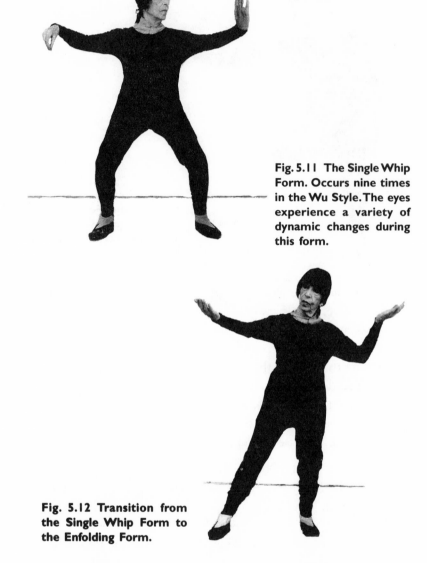

Fig. 5.11 The Single Whip Form. Occurs nine times in the Wu Style. The eyes experience a variety of dynamic changes during this form.

Fig. 5.12 Transition from the Single Whip Form to the Enfolding Form.

and head then gently recover the normal position on the next transition movement. There are several transition movements in which the head is tipped to exercise the muscles in a different and more intense way.

3. The Single Whip Form appears nine times in the Wu style. The eyes experience a variety of dynamic changes which are specially designed for this Form. The eyes follow the movement of the left hand, which travels at shoulder height from the right side to the left side. The eyes follow the path of the hand as it rises and falls. The eye muscles change in slow succession from a relaxed to a tensed state and back to a relaxed state. In passing from the right to the left side, the hand travels in a parabola. The eyes are then activated more tensely as the palm reaches the center of the curve at chest level because the gaze has moved in a downward and inward path. The gaze then moves upward toward the left, releasing eye pressure as the hand completes the movement at the left side, still at shoulder height. Here the eyes see the back of the hand. The eyes have been slowly activated by a relatively light tension and a strong one, and then "released" to become quietly and evenly relaxed at the end of the arm-hand-head movement. (The head is held level as it moves from the right side to the left while the eyes follow the hand (parabola) movement. (Fig. 5-11)

4. The Oblique Look: When the eyes are directed to look far right or left, the head must be slightly tipped downward to avoid extreme pressure on the muscles (as in the Flying Oblique Form explained above). In a transition between the Single Whip Form and the Enfolding Form, the head is tipped on the left side and then moves to off-center right to look obliquely at the right upturned palm, which is at far right. This eye position appears only once, perhaps because it is most tense. The eyes recover their neutral position on the next movement and, relatively speaking, have a "rest" in the basic 45-degree gaze.

Suffice it to say that subtle or obvious eye movements stimulate the agility and the power of the eyes, the movements of which are as necessary to nurture "health and awareness" as are all the other more easily discerned bodily maneuvers.

This analysis encompasses the range of the movements and "stillnesses" of the eye-action: seeing and looking and not commenting or mentally reacting to what is observed. The eyes function as naturally as does every other part of the body, according to the dictates of the mind and the demands of form, direction, space, time, and the dynamic interplay of all these factors.

The eyes become (and remain) intelligent and tranquil and maintain the expressive spirit of the individual personality. They express the essence of T'ai-Chi Ch'uan: calmness, containment, and the comprehension of some possible potential development of consciousness. The Chinese say the eyes are the "cottage of the spirit," the glow of the spirit of equanimity. S. E. Cirlot, in the *Dictionary of Symbols*, says: "Light is symbolic of intelligence and of the spirit. . . . [T]he process of seeing represents a spiritual act and symbolizes understanding."

4. The Quiet Control of the Head

An investigation of things leads to the existence of knowledge.—Chu Hsi (1130–1200 C.E.)

How beautifully assured a person appears to be when the head is placed, held and carried in such a way that the neck and shoulders are at ease. The quiet control of the well-held head depends on the close and immediate assistance of both neck and shoulders to form (with it) unity of action.

No matter whether the head is kept still or whether it moves slightly as in turning, tipping, or lowering, its relationship with the neck and shoulders can be maintained in complete physiological harmony if the dynamics of effort and release are properly balanced.

The neck supporting the head is itself supported by the shoulders. Although it cannot move "independently," the neck is never rigid, tense or constrained, unless the head and shoulder "misbehave," that is, when the shoulders tense awkwardly or the head hangs, loosely dropped downward.

In its self-stillness, the neck can be viewed as being a pillar of strength, adjusting with ease to every head or shoulder motion, or remaining utterly still with equal ease. The muscles of the neck are regulated to react to the demands of form and patterns.

The column of the neck is extremely vulnerable, since it is the pathway for oxygen and blood circulation to the head area and for the swallowing and breathing processes.

Undue pressure on it from a heavily hanging head, for instance, or from a falsely activated shoulder (emotional or physical) constantly and automatically imperils and impairs the basic circulatory processes throughout the entire bodily system.

Therefore, the knowledge of how to move this "three-some"—head, neck, shoulders—in relation to each other is a fundamental requirement for achieving well-being physically and emotionally.

To understand what occurs in the manipulation of each part, singly or in combination, is to reduce the possibility of destructive activity or careless accidents in these regions.

For the head to be in quiet control with ease and authority, the total body must conduct itself with physiological correctness and be supremely able to maintain "awareness" of the quality of its lightness.

I have as yet not mentioned mind—which does not imply that I underestimate the power of its presence. There is nothing without mind accompaniment in T'ai-Chi Ch'uan, the philosophy of which simply states that mind and body must be in accord at all times.

The analysis and illustrations to follow will emphasize the physicality of the relationships of head, neck, and shoulders and explain the influences each has on the others—all of which, I hope, will make evident the necessity of understanding and appreciating what dynamic interchanges take place reciprocally.

The various sections and groupings explain how, when, where, and why the head, neck, and shoulders naturally affect each other—with specific references to movements, positions, and forms as they appear in the Wu style of T'ai-Chi Ch'uan.

Since the exercise is so completely varied, my illustrations may be limited (as well they are!), but they cannot be considered meager, because what is illustrated with clarity in certain formations can be identified elsewhere in the formidable structure by a player who is creative and inspired enough to do so (a most pleasurable and enlightening task!).

To study and experience technically the details of this uniquely composed exercise will not dispel or dampen the spirit of the feeling-sensation to be derived from the "wholeness" of the composition.

On the contrary, the perceptions will enrich one. Just as a musician who cannot render the essence of a musical score without understanding the smallest aspect of tone relationships as they appear in a larger phrase, so the T'ai-Chi Ch'uan player, by setting the mind on what the body does physically in relation to structure, will perceive the great in the little: the "great" (the unity) being the balanced harmony of time-space dynamics-form.

The Basic Body Form

The organic harmony of the entire body form extends from the firm foundation of the foot-leg stance (*shih*, solid) through and to the feathery lightness of the carriage of the head (*hsu*, void).

When the various sections of the body are correctly aligned and therefore are comfortably balanced, the weight of the body is being distributed proportionately to each different part according to need.

The result for a person so well adjusted is a feeling of weightlessness—this is the equivalent of being light. The player will experience such lightness if the detailed coordinated structure is performed with physiological exactness.

It almost goes without saying that the physicality of power (gravity) lies in the pelvic area. The torso rests lightly on the pelvis, almost as if it had no weight; the waist area is free to move agilely.

The frame of the shoulders is held low, pulled down evenly. The neck area is free from any pressure—"empty"—its task (among others) is to hold the head lightly upright. Shoulders properly held will never contract the chest area, nor will they compress the neck muscles. The shoulders, neck, and head, each affecting the other, are held in "vertical" ease.

The spine, straight from base of the skull to the coccyx, is reinforced by the way the buttocks are securely "tucked under"—"not," as Grandmaster Ma Yueh Liang has said, "pushed out like a mountain peak."

The way the head holds itself is the essential fact (and feat) of how to carry oneself at any time, for any task. As the Chinese have so beautifully put it, the head feels as if it were "suspended by silk cord from the heavens." (And what can be more heavenly light than that?) Literally, the head is upright and centered, with the chin level—not lifted or dropped—so that the crown of the head is definitely "facing" vertically upward.

The neck (as will be seen later) reacts to any movements made by either the shoulders or the head. It is remarkable that all responding neck muscle adjustments never affect the larynx, the trachea, or the esophagus regions negatively.

The head can be placed in different positions whether or not the body is in motion; and it can remain utterly still when various parts of the body are in constant activity. But its quiet control depends absolutely on what the shoulders do at all times.

If, for instance, the shoulders pull up tensely toward the ears, thus irritating the neck muscles, the head will feel heavy, awkward, and "disabled." However, the impeccably correct relationships of both neck and shoulders at every instant in T'ai-Chi Ch'uan helps to keep the head in quiet control.

Even when the head changes position it is in quiet control, alert, and attentive. And even then it appears to be still—with an air of authority. Perhaps we can say that awareness of its "presence" controls its quietness.

If awareness of body and head "evaporate," the "abandoned" head will flop and wobble aimlessly—for example, when one falls asleep sitting up, without any head support, the pull of gravity takes over. The mind being "absent," all authority is lost.

Thus, we cannot doubt that it is our mind (mind-will) that helps the head maintain its quiet control, whatever the action and form combinations being made by the total body.

The illustrations to come concentrate on the action of head, neck, and shoulders and the degree to which they affect each other, structurally and dynamically.

The relationships, each to the other, are always balanced in terms of shape, direction, and dynamic yin-yang interplay. All in diverse ways contribute to the experience of being centered, light, and calm—and also to being in quiet control.

Analysis of the Structural Relationships of Head, Neck, and Shoulder Movements

The head will always be in quiet control, no matter how intricate the movements made by the neck, shoulders, and the head itself.

It is not visually obvious that the neck area is greatly affected both by every change of head position and by the variations in shoulder motion. The neck responds to even the very slightest action above it and below it, the degree of muscular tension depending on the kind of movement causing it.

The analysis of what physical reactions take place in neck and/or shoulders to maintain the head in quiet control can be put into two main categories of movements:

(I.) When Head Remains Still; and (II.) When the Head Moves.

I. When the Head Remains Still

   A. During action of changing forms, where shoulders remain in place.

   B. During action where torso, neck, shoulders are activated for the form positions.

II. When the Head Moves

   A. Changing position where total body remains still.

   B. Changing positions in combination with body movements.

   C. Changing positions in a complex sequence of body movements.

(illustrations are taken from the Wu style).

I.   When the Head Remains Still

    A.   During action of changing forms where shoulders remain in place, unmoving.

      1. In the simplified Walking Step, the entire body goes through many different positions—moving forward or retreating—with torso; legs and arms in constant motion. The head remains still, never stirs out of its straight elevated form. Whether the torso is at slant or vertical, the shoulders also have not been moved out of position. (Form: Brush Knee Twist Step.) (Fig. 5.13.)

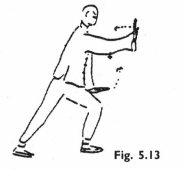
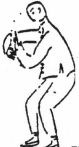

Fig. 5.13   **Fig. 5.14**

      2. When the torso bends forward from the waist at a 45-degree angle, the head does not fall forward. The head and neck retain their basic positions. The relationship of head, neck, and shoulders has remained the same as it was when torso was held vertically. (Form: Step Up—Enfolding Form). (Fig. 5.14.)

      3. Standing on left leg with the other leg raised up in an angled position; the torso bends forward from the waist (a 45-degree angle); arms are curved, the left fist near forehead and the right elbow rests on raised right knee—the head, neck and shoulders do not change their relationships of the basic posture. (Form: Beat the Tiger.) (Fig. 5.15.)

      4. When the torso, "sitting" on the right leg with bent knee (in the Empty Step), is on a diagonal slant forward, with

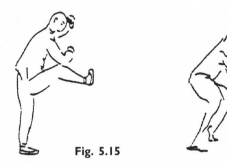

Fig. 5.15   Fig. 5.16

the right arm outstretched and "tensed," head, neck, and shoulders remain still. (Form: The Golden Needle at the Bottom of the Deep Sea.) (Fig. 5.16.)

5. In swift moving Forms or Transitions (there are nine in Wu style) the head, neck, and shoulders retain their "quiet" relationships, never moving out of place while executing the swift form.

One of the most difficult of the nine places where this occurs is the Lotus Swing Form where arms must slap a fast-moving right leg swinging in an elevated arc. The head is in quiet control, as the torso bends forward with the action. Neck and shoulders do not stir out of place. (Fig. 5.17.)

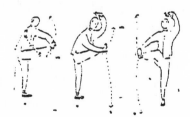

Fig. 5.17

B. When head remains still, in place, while shoulders and/ or torso change positions and directions.

1. From the Parry Form, the right hand (fisted) moves to the lower right hip side, with the elbow sharply angled to point to right side—out, away from the torso. The placement of the right fist at the right hip, while keeping the right elbow out to the right, causes the right shoulder to contract (yang contraction).

This movement forces the neck muscles on right side to react tensely. The left side of neck remains light. Neither the left shoulder nor the neck has moved. The head stays still in quiet control. (Fig. 5.18.)

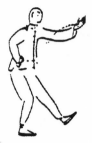

Fig. 5.18

2. Position: Torso, head, and arm are directed toward the corner of the room, that is, at a 45-degree angle from a front position. The right arm is shoulder high, bent at the elbow which is a "squared" or 90-degree angle; the right palm horizontally faces the left shoulder.

The left palm, with fingers vertical, is crossed near the right palm, close to it; the left elbow is low at the left side. The head is centered on the quiet shoulders.

Movement: Stirring the right elbow to move right, the torso moves and turns (is drawn) to the front (of room), then to the diagonal right corner, as elbow continues to move to finish out, in line with right shoulder; the elbow has remained bent.

The head has remained still; facing diagonally left during the action, which includes the left arm moving straight to left diagonal.

The head then "sees" the back of the left hand. The action of the torso toward the right has stirred the neck muscles to react because head has remained "in place."

Position precedes Form: Fan Behind the Back. (Fig. 5.19.)

Note: IB.1—Illustrates single shoulder movement affecting neck.

IB.2—Illustrates torso changes affecting neck where the shoulders do not move out of place.

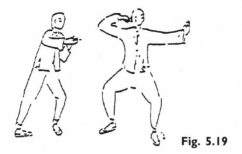

Fig. 5.19

II. When the Head Moves

A. Head changes position while the body does not move.

1. Form: Parting the Wild Horse's Mane (third position). The body is aslant toward the right in an open bow and arrow (leg) form, with torso turned at a 45-degree angle toward the front. Right arm is extended toward right direction at shoulder level.

Movement: Head moves to the right shoulder side, activating the neck muscles, while the rest of body remains still. (In the Form to follow [IB], the head remains still; the action of the torso returns to a position which will release the tension of the neck muscles.) (Fig. 5.20.)

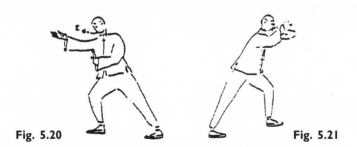

Fig. 5.20   **Fig. 5.21**

2. Position: Body is in Walking Stance. Head looks directly forward. Both hands are fisted; wrists are crossed at left side just above left shoulder level.

Elbows are shoulder high. This Form make right-shoulder contract, affecting neck muscles on right side while left side is quiet. (Fig. 5.21.)

Movement: Head moves toward right shoulder, keeping level, thus intensifying the neck muscles on left side.

In this position, there is a double tension: (1) when the shoulder action affects the neck; and (2) when the head action directs the neck. (Form: precedes the position of Right Open Leg lift.) (Fig. 5.21.)

> B. Head changes positions in combination with body movements.

1. Completing the Single Whip Form: Movements of legs, arms, torso, and also eyes are being made while the head turns. Movement: keeping level, the head moves from the right side to the left shoulder side.

The neck muscles are activated and tensed when the head is turned from right to left; and with firmer tension when the head is turned to complete the left-sided movement.

There is reduced tension when the head passes through the "centered" position between the shoulders, which do not move out of place. This movement occurs nine times in the Wu style. (Fig. 5.22.)

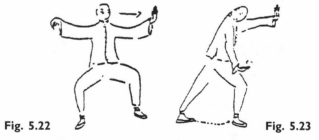

Fig. 5.22   **Fig. 5.23**

2. Position: A Walking Stance, with right leg front and left leg straight behind; right palm faces downward in front of right knee; head is level and centered.

Movement: Three movements are done at the same time: (1) head tips downward, with chin turned toward right side; the face is therefore a-slant; eyes look downward as (2) right palm turns upward; (3) right foot is angled 45-degrees toward the front of room. Back and side muscles of neck are activated. Form: Beginning of Flying Oblique. (Fig. 5.23.)

C. Head changes positions consecutively in combination with other movements.

1. Position: From the Form of the Single Whip stance (IIB), the head is looking left at the left hand; the right arm is outstretched toward the right; the body is in a Horseback Riding stance.

Movement: Head, arms, legs, torso all move in combination toward the Enfolding Form (IA.2)

The head tips downward on left side, turns toward front, and then moves toward the right; eyes can see right hand; head remains tipped and "a-slant."

Legs are being adjusted, as are arms to move into the basic front stance of the Enfolding Form—while this action is taking place, the head moves into its basic light position (IA.2). The neck has been activated throughout, with shoulders not moving. (Fig. 5.24.)

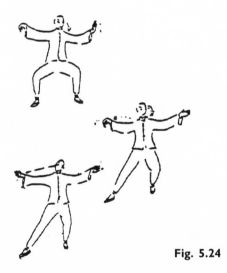

Fig. 5.24

Note the wave of changing dynamics in the neck. The quality of quiet control has not been lost during this complex movement. This illustration of complex head-movements is similar, with variations, to dozens of others. Awareness of the "delicacy" of the changes protects the quality of quiet control.

Of necessity, I have given only a few examples of the many which are intrinsically similar to those described. It must, however, be emphasized and reiterated that no two actions are ever exactly the same, since the ingredients of any movement may be subtly different as to tempo, space-action, quality, direction, and the connective sequences.

Nevertheless, the player will be led to discover and perceive the inevitability of the dynamic connections of various parts of the body physically, from the above examples; and will also begin to discern and appreciate the body's innate powers to respond to the complexity of manmade (mind's) creative thinking.

The technique becomes absorbed in the balanced process of body and mind harmoniousness. The spirit will never disappear despite deep study of what creates it.

It is to be noted that 90 percent of the time during which the action is passing from one part of the body to some other with dynamics and forms in ever-changing related harmonies, the head has accompanied the movements with the poised presence of stillness.

Although separate head movements consciously directed to fit the form are relatively few, they contribute profoundly not only to the physical welfare of the system but also to the aesthetics and spirit of T'ai-Chi Ch'uan.

As the head moves into the rare and difficult positions, it is with a control equal to the intrinsic "effort" necessary to keep the head still. It can be considered the yang quality (II A, B, C above) of the moving structure in balanced relativity to the yin quality of no-movement (I A, B).

A deep feeling of serenity settles into the heart of the player when the exercise is performed with meaningful form and the mindful spirit of the "Quiet Control of the Head."

5. Some Distinguishing Features of the Wu and Yang Styles

Time and time again I have been asked in what respects the Yang and Wu styles of T'ai-Chi Ch'uan differ, both being of the intrinsic (*nei jia*) school for activating the body for the development of physical, emotional, and mental well-being.

The Wu Chien Ch'uan style is the descendant, as it were, of the Yang Lu-Ch'an style, which in turn is a variation of the Chen style. Each style is named for its "creative" master.

The reasons for creative changes, constructive variations or additions come from the basic philosophic attitude of each "profound" master toward the increased possibilities of developing enduring physical prowess with mental control of intricate coordination, and with greater demands on both body and mind to achieve a more profound state of self-"being," physically and spiritually.

In the Wu style (of which I am an ardent exponent), a keener "telescopic" eye and mind (like discovering a "new" star) helped to give T'ai-Chi Ch'uan more subtle structural relationships—as, for instance, adding more minute movements to larger ones to improve physical power and mental awareness.

Both Are Consistent in Form

Clarity of vision and clarity of purpose create, as Grandmaster Ma Yueh-liang told me, a "flowering" on a higher plane, enriching the basic creations of the past.

Both Yang and Wu styles are each impeccably consistent in form, function, and long-term goals. Each style has 108 Forms (therefore there are 108 Transitions which connect them).

The technical movement is continuous and flowing in slow tempo (heartbeat time); all strive for balance, stability, and harmony. Above all, the mind is always present to direct action.

No extraneous tenseness-hardness is allowed; all movements are intrinsically dynamic; yin and yang, *hsu* (void) and *shih* (weighted) changes are results of the physiologically patterned action.

The following analysis of some of the positions, movements, and physiological techniques exemplify, on an obvious level (those which can be easily recognized), how and where Wu and Yang differ. Each one is a fundamentally characteristic feature.

1. Basic Stance (at the beginning)

Wu style:

Feet are placed one foot length apart with feet parallel forming a square basic stance. Legs are therefore parallel.

Yang style:

Feet are placed apart slightly wider than a square with toes turned out slightly. Legs are therefore separated at a slight diagonal. (Fig. 5.25.)

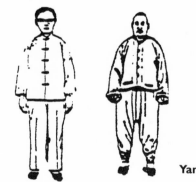

Wu   Yang

Fig. 5.25 The Basic Stances

2. The Single Whip

Wu style:

Legs are separated, with feet (heels) two foot-lengths apart; toes turned outward slightly (or they may be kept parallel). Both knees are equally bent. Arms are diagonally forward at shoulder height. Torso is centered; the stance is symmetrical. The head is turned to the left; and the hand positions are different. (Fig. 5.26.)

Yang style:

Legs are separated; weight is on left leg with bent knee; right knee is straight. Therefore weight is mostly on the left side. Left arm is slightly higher than shoulder; head and hands are positioned as in Wu style. (Fig. 5.27.)

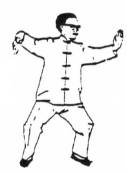 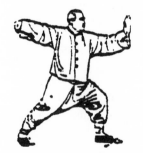

Fig. 5.26 Wu Single Whip   **Fig. 5.27 Yang Single Whip**

3. Brush Knee Twist Step (The Walking Step)

Wu style:

Front knee is bent and rear leg is straight and firm from hip. Feet are about eighteen inches apart; front foot always points in the direction required; rear foot "tries" to be parallel to it. When rear leg advances the front foot remains in its position. The torso faces the direction of the front foot and is a-slant; head to rear heel are in a spine-straight diagonal.

Yang style:

Legs are similarly (as above) apart but with rear toe turned out 45 degrees; and rear knee is bent—thus keeping the torso vertical. More weight is on front leg. Before advancing, the front foot is turned "outward" 45 degrees. Then the rear leg is placed forward with toe pointing in the required direction. Therefore, in this Form there is an angled rear foot advancing the straight front foot.

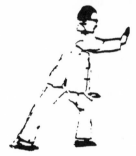 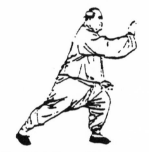

Fig. 5.28 Wu Brush Knee Twist Step   **Fig. 5.29 Yang Brush Knee Twist Step**

4. Traveling in the Walking Step

Wu style:

In bringing the rear leg to step forward, the heel is raised thus bending the knee. The leg is then brought forward so that the toe just misses touching the floor, with the foot "hanging" loosely, after which it is flexed for the "empty" foot position.

Yang style:

In bringing the rear leg forward the knee is lifted up high, thus raising the leg far up from the ground.

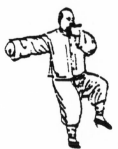

Fig. 5.30 Yang Walking with High Step

Wu style:

Leg position: The right raised leg is held high so that the knee is positioned at a 130-degree angle. Therefore, the lower part of the leg is angled obliquely forward. In all the leg lift forms with high knee, the leg takes the same 130-degree angled position.

Yang style:

The right leg is held so that the lower part hangs vertically forming a 90-degree angle at the knee.

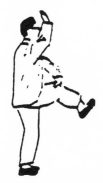

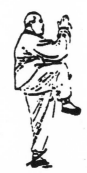

Fig. 5.31 Wu Golden Cockerel on One Leg

Fig. 5.32 Yang Golden Cockerel on One Leg

6. Arms

Wu style:

Arms have wide range of space-movement from full out to close to body, with a great variety of movements in between. The clarity of the combination of the arc (circle) gesture coordinated with the wavelike (elbow-wrist-hand) position is extremely important structurally and physiologically.

Yang style:

There is a full range of expanding circular movements, but (to my knowledge) there are fewer variations of closer arm-wrist-elbow forms.

7. Hands-Wrists-Fingers

Wu style:

The wrist movement and hand shape are greatly diversified, emphasizing the yin-yang action of dynamics and space-directions, every minute change significantly formed.

Yang style:

Hand forms are less diverse, with the wrist less active and the play of hand changes less varied than in Wu.

8. The Nine Speedy Extrinsic Movements (each different from the other)

Wu style:

These were taught to me as being important to develop quick reflexes; to be able to go from slow to speedy and vice versa in a fraction of a second, indicating complete concentration and physical prowess. (Useful of course in the application of self-defense activity.)

Yang style:

In China I never saw any "fast" movements in this structure.

9. The Number of "Series" (Divisions)

Wu style:

There are six series in the total composition which can be analyzed physically, structurally, and philosophically. None, however, show their endings or beginnings.

Each series is a stage in self-development as one advances in understanding the harmony of T'ai-Chi Ch'uan and as one experiences its spirit in terms of patience, tranquility, insight, and awareness on more profound levels.

Yang style:

The composition is "divided" into three series. I do not know the reasons for this division.

10. Comments

What matters, ultimately, for all the long Ch'uan—Chen, Yang, Wu, Sun, Ho (and others somewhere perhaps?)—are not the differences, but the profound equivalents. All move on the same paths for achieving knowledge and the experience of what constitutes a harmonious personality for balanced healthfulness and longevity.

The drawings for this article were taken from "Wu Style Taichichuan," by Wu Ying-hua and Ma Yueh-liang and "Tai-chi Chuan," by Yearning K. Chen, Yang Style.

6. The Exercise-Art as It Functions Creatively for the Actor

An actor in Shanghai's Classical Chinese Theater, Wang Fu-Ying (my instructor in the Chinese Theater's dance-roles), said to me: "We actors all do T'ai-Chi Ch'uan every day. It functions as a great medium for stabilizing health and who needs more body-and-mind health than an actor who must expend so much energy." I had had, at the time, a few months of lessons with Mr. Ma Yueh-Liang, the eminent master of T'ai-Chi Ch'uan. Those lessons impressed me with the singularity of the art; it has no drama and no personal emotions, and is directed to the *self* and not to an audience, as acting is.

At the Actors' Studio in New York an actor said to me, after a dozen lessons in T'ai-Chi Ch'uan, "What a difference I now feel between getting somewhere and 'the going' there, as, for instance, in moving from one side of the stage to the other. Now I do not just get there mindlessly, but I can be 'with myself' in the going. I'm sure this awareness further extended offers many possibilities for dramatic action."

A director remarked, "I can see how the remarkable uses of personal dynamics, intrinsically felt, with directional changes of body-form and space-form, can be augmented and developed to manipulate actors on stage with more vital, varied, visual complexities."

The actor, with growing sensitivity, was able to apply *the way* of movement to a practical situation, and had acquired the attentiveness of mind to "be with" the less tangible connective links natural to any series of gestures, ordinarily ignored. He was beginning to enrich his role with added consciousness and technical proficiency. The director was thinking creatively of architectural form, visualizing a dynamic structure in terms of counter-forces, body and space relationships, as he himself acquired the concepts of the composition through doing it.

Not only is T'ai-Chi Ch'uan a process for personal improvement, but it is also a creative stimulus for specialized skills, and applicable in a multitude of imaginative ways to whatever one's interests are. Awareness of what is, and the knowledge of how to change what is, is intrinsic to the harmonious system of T'ai-Chi Ch'uan, an ancient Chinese exercise-art (said to have been perfected c. 1100 C.E.).

Not mime, not dance, not an acting craft, T'ai-Chi Ch'uan is a complete exercise-technique. Ch'uan (as simply stated by Chinese writers) is "to move hands, arms, elbows, shoulders, palms, fists, legs, knees, feet, toes, waist, torso, neck, head, eyes in harmonious combinations systematically arranged," all designed with intricate variations and balanced unity. It is the philosophic and scientific *way* of T'ai-Chi Ch'uan which determines how the interacting forces of yin and yang (light-strong, empty-solid, quiet-active) function and which forms the dynamic structure. With *the way* of movement light, even, slow, continuous, and in balance, attention is alerted to the most minute detail and emotional security is attained, and because neither the heartbeat nor breath is speeded up during even the most complicated action, physical efficiency is increased.

T'ai-Chi Ch'uan has no stylistic mannerisms, a fact which is extremely important (for the actor): styled exercising technique superimposes a point of view, limits further expressiveness, and colors characterizations. This Chinese exercise system is natural to the "nth" degree, built as it is on the

fundamental physiological laws that control human behavior
in all its complex variety, and thus frees the personality and
reveals its potentialities by making it more adaptable, versatile,
and pliable.

T'ai-Chi Ch'uan, unlike any other known exercise, is especially unusual (among many other reasons) in the fact of its
length—that it lasts twenty-two to twenty-five minutes without
stopping in a continuously flowing series of interconnected movements. It is *one* exercise, a long composition of 108 Forms, complicatedly, artfully, and scientifically connected so that the patterns
move from one part of the body to another without strain and
without overworking a single part: complicatedly—to develop coordination and concentration; artfully—to sustain one's interest
and to make the mind participate in the action: scientifically—to
develop stamina, endurance, and efficiency as well as to correct
defects. This unbroken *oneness* creates an immense capacity to
persevere with patience, with increasingly sustained energy.

No emotion, or whatever is called self-expression, motivates the movement. The feeling is that of *being,* which not only
produces poise, but actually raises the level of vitality. The sensation is that of *well-being* which produces a state of calmness, a
settled state of mind (the Chinese word for heart and mind
being the same). Despite this impersonality and objective self-discipline, T'ai-Chi Ch'uan becomes a very intimate and personal matter with each one, as the process of self-discovery begins
to put one at ease with oneself and gives one the assurance of
one's personality.

The complete exercise is a unity of changing action,
functional on every level, impressive in its variety. The ingredients of form and direction, space and time, light and strong (yin-yang) dynamics present even in the smallest patterned groups
are so organically intertwined as to be the very warp and woof
of this "symphonic" composition. The interrelated qualities, essential equally to the structure and the way of movement, can
be characterized as follows:

1. *Soft-intrinsic:* No extra pressure or tension is used to execute a movement, beyond what is necessary to effect it. "To lift a pound, use only that much force." This is built-in or intrinsic-to-the-need energy, as a result of which the appearance is soft (which is not flabbiness). Softness results from the perfect balance of physical content (muscularization) with the form-structure. No matter how much stress the action requires, there is never any tensed expenditure of energy beyond necessity. A "reserve of energy like a bow about to be snapped" adds to the accumulation of powerful resources and counteracts tenseness.

2. *Slow:* The tempo is so natural that since neither the heartbeat nor breathing is quickened, stamina is stored up and patience naturally increases.

3. *Connected and flowing:* All action is consistently connected "like a series of pleats, folding in on itself with rhythm and order." The flowing aspect eliminates any break between form and movement. With such action, it is possible to experience calmness and serenity.

4. *Continuous:* Unceasing motion throughout the entire twenty-two to twenty-five minute exercise develops great endurance and potential power, with control and heightened awareness.

5. *Balance:* The adjustment of dynamics with the structural forms is so exact that "a feather cannot be added nor a fly land without effecting a change," so mathematically correct is the intrinsic form, so sensitized is the performer. Disciplined control of balance over the force of gravity inevitably improves coordination and body harmony. A sense of balance necessarily refers to a state of mind as well.

6. *Dynamics:* From the most subtle lightness to the point of strength just short of final power the dynamics of the

exercise is in continuous alternation in all possible nuances (yin-yang). "Like the flowing movement of a river"
which would not move unless there were variations of
energy and release, so the body itself is released with
many dynamic changes. This changing aspect of the T'ai-
Chi Ch'uan is most basic in keeping in balance the circulatory and respiratory systems and also in preventing
fatigue. This regularly maintained "undulation" of forces
makes the body flexible, resilient, and dexterous.

7. *Circular:* Movement (in arcs, spirals, parabolas, ovals,
   etc.) in contrast to hard-edged linear gestures, keeps the
   body from expending itself and contributes to the feeling of security and containment.

8. *The mind:* The participating mind is always present to
   direct the action; because of this "from the mind attention," alertness is enhanced, power of observation and
   perceptivity increased. "Attention is centered not only
   on the fixed gestures but on the movements changing
   from one to the other." When the mind is both the
   instigator and the observer, as "the mind directs the
   energy and the energy exercises the body," mental blank-
   outs, absentmindedness, and automatic behavior can
   never occur.

9. *Active and still:* Throughout the perpetual movement
   there is in each Form some part of the body which is
   nonmoving and quiet, as if it were a point of reference
   from which comes a feeling of alert attention, "like the
   spirit of a cat waiting to catch a mouse." From subtle
   combinations of cause and effect, of quiet and active, is
   developed a more profound ability to control complex
   situations.

10. *Complex:* The multiplicity of postures, designs, themes,
    and Forms with their interweaving patterns exercises the
    entire body internally and externally. The very variety

keeps interest from flagging. To learn and perform these combinations demands and develops concentration, improves coordination, increases attentiveness, and makes the mind's will overcome the inertia of the body. Aesthetically satisfying, the varied structure in time and space, direction and form, essence and quality is stimulating as an art experience.

As a specific example of the complexity of a Form, let me describe the action of Cloud Arms, a Form which (as do all) exemplifies the intricate way the torso, joints, and spine behave when combinations of pattern and design motivate the activity. You will note that no *single group* of muscles are stirred in "isolation" in a one-and-two beat, as happens in other exercise techniques, where, as for instance, arms are swung to and fro, or bodies moved up and down, with elementary rhythm and without "reference" to each other, and with no structural significance.

Every one of the 108 Forms is total in concept. Each contains some action for most of the Body, in differing sequences and designs, and with varying degrees of emphasis on *all* the above-mentioned qualities found in T'ai-Chi Ch'uan as a whole.

Whatever takes place in the complete exercise is both the seed and the result of other action, each dovetailing, joining, and overlapping with other units. This gives the player a great feeling of being *in* a composition and of *being* it because he himself, aware of his own being, seems to be the cause of it. T'ai-Chi Ch'uan is so integrated with respect to itself and to the one who "plays" it that the benefits can even creep in on him unwittingly; he cannot be other than affected by the participation of both his body and his brain. But when he is in command of himself, then he begins to be a sentient being, synthesizing the acts of doing, knowing, and being.

More than in any other profession, the actor must not only *be* but must have within him the ability to *become*, not merely to play a part, but to become it. He must be able to capture the totality of a part in movement, rhythm, voice, emotion and reproduce a coordinated personality without any interference from his clearly defined private one.

To perform in any theater of no matter what style— New, Classic, Absurd, or the Happening variety (where even without having an acting part, the person, to say the least, must *be* someone to control his identity)—the actor must have initiative, inventiveness, and adaptability; a capacity to feel and respond, to change and simulate, to become; the capability to observe, experience, and imagine, to emphasize and create. Such assurance of self cannot come about except with a penetrating knowledge of how the body behaves under all conditions, and how to make it take on meaning, how to relate to the enacted personality, and also to know when and how to abandon it and not continue to play the stage-framed role at the coffee-counter.

T'ai-Chi Ch'uan can be of use as a constructive means to a self-expressive end (one's profession) or, as a constructive end in itself, be a means for the expression of the self. Because this exercise-art is so astutely integrated for use in life, the nature of its composite forms being organic and natural as applied to mental and physical development, and because its profoundly subtle structure centers the mind and calms the emotions, its physical techniques and practical concepts can be applied to the theatrical arts, which comprise a small universe in themselves. Within the boundaries of the actor's art, the following briefly summarizes some of the vital elements which can enhance the actor's vitality by doing and getting-to-know-himself through the practice of T'ai-Chi Ch'uan.

Although the physical, emotional, and mental results evolve simultaneously from a given situation, I nevertheless separate them for reasons of clarity and convenience. Physically speaking, excluding the enumeration of healthful improvements, one will be able to manipulate the body for any desired effect without abusing it; the voice can be improved through better capacity for breathing properly and correct posture, with no strain in neck or shoulders; the body will move with ease and harmony under *any* condition, and will be agile and flexible; one will be able, with a greater capacity for work without tiring, to do more with less expenditure of energy and to be in control of one's dynamic tensions.

Regarding the emotional aspect, self-consciousness disappears through self-control; stage nerves can be quickly obliterated by the act of doing even a *part* of the exercise; an easier disposition, balanced temperament, and patience become part of one's nature, as does the capacity to persevere. One can quickly detect one's own indisposition and overcome it, can remain imperturbable in disagreeable situations, and, becoming astute regarding others' motivations, one can take criticism with equanimity.

And regarding the mental aspect, interests are heightened, which in itself is healthy: new insights can make one more creative and enhance characterizations; the ability to memorize rapidly with easy concentration is improved; awareness of self and of others enlarges one's capacity to observe; rapid reflexes result in greater dexterity in doing and learning, which then become part of living; everything falls into place when the mind can ignore irrelevant problems. The discerning mind perceives the organic and inevitable consequences of movement, and so the possibilities for new relationships and combinations are creatively widened.

That this list of beneficial results is not exaggerated can be attested by anyone who has begun to appreciate the immensity of the scope—philosophical and practical—of T'ai-Chi Ch'uan, evolved over the centuries by men of thought who were also men of action, and by men of action who were also philosophers.

I now return, like the T'ai-Chi symbol, circling on itself with calm certitude, to the beginning, where I spoke of this art as being directed to the *self* rather than to an audience. The art of the theater, like any of the fine arts, is designed to stimulate the hearts and minds of the audience, to be, so to speak, participated in and "completed" by the spectators' reactions. T'ai-Chi Ch'uan is an art for the practitioner, who receives the total benefits of the physical, emotional, and mental efforts. This difference is essential to the appreciation of this exercise as a personal art. However, as yin and yang mutually aid each other, the art for the practitioner who is an actor will eventually benefit his audience through the medium of the actor's improved skills and creative, stable personality.

CHAPTER VI

THE INTRINSIC LOGIC OF PHILOSOPHY

Action uncoils, interlacing
Shape to form, reshaping time and space.
Flowing, rolling on with force inside—
Gentleness outside like water spreading
Down a shallow slope persuasively
Filling crevices with nonchalance,
Designing forms and changing course
According to the nature
Of the changing situation
  Waving-curving, arcing-circling,
  Ebbing-flowing, immense or small,
  From obvious to delicate,
  The T'ai-Chi Way of Movement
  Fits the Forms of Being
  In every subtle turn and minute spot,
  Dynamics interplaying
  Alternating with the nature
    Of the changes changing.   167

The Intrinsic Logic of Philosophy

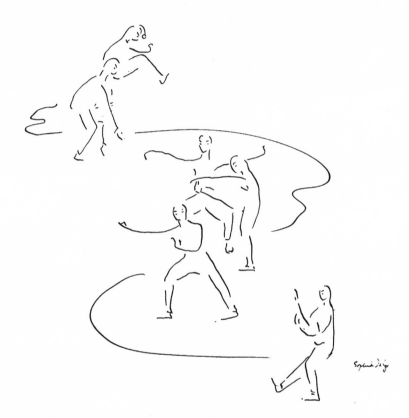

Harmonious Diversity

1. A Harmony of Change

Embedded in the very nature of T'ai-Chi Ch'uan is the principle that every aspect of its continually moving process must be harmonious. This principle, the essence of mind-body equilibrium, directs the content, organizes the form, and diversifies the motion so that all becomes a harmony of change in balanced proportions.

Just as organic matter is in a state of continual change and motion, so the manmade exercise of T'ai-Chi Ch'uan is an image of nature's fundamental way. The T'ai-Chi Ch'uan changes have been made harmonious by men and women's understanding of their own natures and by their optimistic belief in the possibility of continual development on higher planes of self-knowledge.

Such harmony presumes the refined interaction of the physical and mental, the instinctive and the psychological, with the organized and organic principles of the T'ai-Chi—the philosophical way, and of the Ch'uan—the physical way. Harmony is the intrinsic relationship of all the structure's qualities intercontrolled.

Harmony at every part of the moving whole is felt at each "caught" moment of the configurations which balance space, position, energy, weight, and lightness. Harmony is felt at every motion in the forming patterns as each subtly connects with what follows in terms of physiology and in terms of the eight directions of space.

Simultaneous as a chord in music, each separate patterned T'ai-Chi Ch'uan form is a single chord of action. T'ai-Chi Ch'uan, as a complete exercise, can be considered a *total* chord in the light of it having attained the integration of meaning and method.

T'ai-Chi Ch'uan becomes a highly complex synthesis which is the result of harmonious fusion of the multiplicity of changing elements balanced at every stage of the exercise's involved activity.

To be aware of the multiplicity of change does not disturb the mind, nor does it distract the self from being centered to attend to the differentiations. Instead, it develops acute sensibility and the mature ability to perceive the *wholeness* as being more significant than the many-shaded combinations within it. Because all changes are created to move consistently and organically in terms of gravity, the dynamic (yin-yang) use of energy is harmonious with the ever-progressing process of change.

With mind in control, the physical body is propelled willingly, smoothly, and flowingly from one movement to another without any emotion interfering with or influencing even the most subtle unit.

Nonetheless, rising spontaneously, a "feeling" response appears, clear and definite, which can be described as a sensing of the harmonious nature of what is being enacted at all times. Agreeable, comforting, calming, with a glow of satisfaction—this is the composite and the pervasive feeling. When body and mind function in unity continually, this initial feeling, this pleasurable reaction, is gradually transformed into a higher state—that of containment, secure and serene.

As a "philosophy" of physical discipline integrating mind-feeling with the nurturing of the internal/external bodily system, T'ai-Chi Ch'uan unites *all* (changes) into *one* (harmony) and thus succeeds in making oneness of all, a harmony of change.

2. The Spirit of Adventure in T'ai-Chi Ch'uan

For both the beginner and the experienced player of T'ai-Chi Ch'uan, this harmonious exercise will be and can continue to be an adventure—an adventure in discovering how to function through life with mental ease, emotional equanimity, and physical well-being.

Whatever the level of experience, the player will continually meet up with, and often be surprised by, some new aspect of the art, discovering features hitherto unsuspected. This provides further insight to the depths of the substance of the exercises in relation to personal progress. The greater the experience the richer is the field for discovery—as more and more of the structure's intricacies touch the attention of the player.

One facet of the adventure in doing T'ai-Chi Ch'uan is the increasing ability to concentrate on the structured action without ever anticipating or planning for the results beforehand. Yet another facet is to see the dynamics of the activity in the terms of space and time; another is in the development of physical security and stamina. Yet another dimension is to be able to maintain the quiescence of torso and head. The harmony of the form and movement produces these results, which are contained in the nature of T'ai-Chi Ch'uan. They will reveal themselves gradually as the player senses and experiences the essence of what being enacted.

In contrast to the T'ai-Chi Ch'uan method of how the goals (not formulated in advance) are achieved, I offer an example of the adventure a mountain climber undergoes. Knowledge of the goal and the way to attain it are clear: to reach the summit of a particular mountain and literally to touch its peak. The ascent produces the adventure and becomes the spirit of the adventure: to overcome and endure whatever unsuspected hardships arise. The climber is relatively prepared for an immense variety of unpleasant situations like snow, wind, tempests, altitude, and difficult terrain. The great adventure is the peak; this goal is ever in mind. (Perhaps without unexpected difficulties it would not be considered an adventure!)

With T'ai-Chi Ch'uan, the ultimate goals are not "visible" materially or mentally, and cannot even be comprehended, aside from an intellectual acquaintance with certain words like calmness, containment, and heightened consciousness—toward which T'ai-Chi Ch'uan is directed.

The player has no idea of when those agreeable qualities will appear and is therefore not concerned in advance about feeling them. What will be born or comes to light depends entirely on the player's prowess, sensitivity, and ability to render and understand the organized composition of T'ai-Chi Ch'uan, which, no matter what, will always nudge the player into some kind of awareness of a very personal feeling of complete ease. This is where the adventure lies: in sensing and experiencing the unity of this complex composition in which the goals are embedded and ready to be exposed.

The journey of T'ai-Chi Ch'uan is comprised of an organic physiological technique that requires complete mental cooperation, the balanced harmony of which (mind-body) incorporates the individual goals and the composite purpose, which are:

1. Stability, stamina, endurance—every step of the way.

2. Patience arising from concentration on all aspects of action.

3. Perception coming from attending to the smallest detail.

4. Energy from the correct manipulation of intrinsic variations of strength and lightness, therefore never expending energy needlessly.

5. Quickened reflexes from the subtle ability to coordinate.

6. Regular heartbeat and even breathing from obeying the nature of function and form.

7. Calmness of spirit from smooth, continuous movement.

8. All adds up to well-being and ease.

9. Each quality appears gradually (together or separately) during the assiduous practice of T'ai-Chi Ch'uan, progressing to heightened consciousness.

The player will discern, now and then, here and there, in many different places on this complex path, the harmony of the self in action without willing or wishing it—results growing and becoming entrenched in the player's personality. This is the great adventure—not knowing in advance—but recognizing the intrinsic transformations. The player has created the goals— or simply unsheathed them—when the time was ripe for them to appear.

T'ai-Chi Ch'uan continues to be an adventure, on many planes to detect and become sensitive to one's gradual progress (to heights unknown) toward the peaks of self-development. With less and less difficulty, goals are reached, but never without the appearance of newer sparks of comprehension and experiences. The adept player will have good health and promising longer life with body-mind-spirit balance.

The mountain climber revels in the triumphant adventure and in the accomplishment of having reached the goal. The T'ai-Chi Ch'uan player centers on the process—the path—and delights in it, from which the goal is grasped and takes for granted that, with deeper experience, something extraordinary may happen.

The mountain climber knows the nature of his adventure, but does not know absolutely that he will succeed in attaining the goal. When we first embark on T'ai-Chi Ch'uan we do not expect it to be an adventure. Nevertheless, inevitably, some degree of success (that is, goals) will always come, without any preknowledge of what it is to be.

Many adventures come to an end—except perhaps in memory. T'ai-Chi Ch'uan's adventure remains a continuously living one—an adventure of discovery of one's self-development as each stage of experience leads to the realization of another one, with coherent and stable equilibrium. The closer one gets to each conscious stage, the more T'ai-Chi Ch'uan has to offer. Success is implicit in the art (and the science) of T'ai-Chi Ch'uan.

3. Two Portraits of the Exercise-Art of T'ai-Chi Ch'uan
As the Viewer Sees It
As the Player Lives It

Introductory Note

Since T'ai-Chi Ch'uan is a system of exercise for self-development—physically, emotionally, and mentally—there is clearly no need for the presence of a viewer or an audience to react to the exercise-art. However, people do "look-in" on it, as it is being played in a public area or when it is being demonstrated to inform others of its existence. T'ai-Chi Ch'uan is so magnetic that the viewer cannot but have a strong reaction to it. It is this viewpoint and, in contrast, the player's experience of what happens internally that I present here.

The concepts comprising the duo-picture, in juxtaposition, are:

1. No Mind vs. Mind Is Master

2. No Effort vs. All Is a Balance of Effort

3. No Dynamic Changes vs. Constant Variations in Dynamic Tensions

4. Uniformity vs. Nothing Repeats Itself

5. The Surface Softness vs. The Hidden Energy

6. Empty-Minded vs. Centered and Concentrated

7. Detachment vs. Deep Involvement

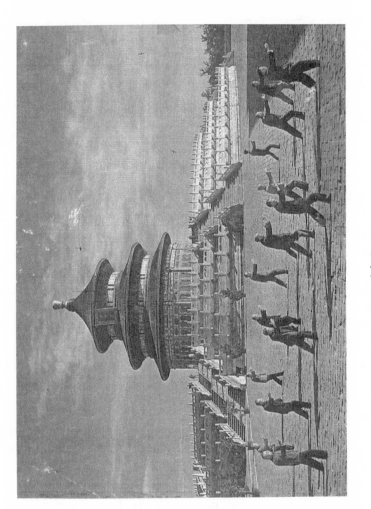

Peaceful Activity

8. Simplicity vs. Multiplicity

9. The Ending Mirrors the Beginning vs. At Completion a New Beginning

As the Viewer Sees It

The picture of T'ai-Chi Ch'uan from the point of view of one who sees it being played is an outline of structural motion framing the figure of the active person who makes the exercise visible in space and time. In addition to the physicality of the form, the viewer's emotional response colors the portrait with the personal feeling of being at ease and calm.

Beautifully visible are the features of the external portrait:

1. No Mind:

An ever changing series of lines and patterns meeting and parting, flowing one into the other spontaneously—as if with no thought or working plan.

As the Player Lives It

The portrait of T'ai-Chi Ch'uan, as the player lives and experiences it, is a multidimensional composition, an intrinsically motivated structure in which the internally felt dynamic interplay of energy and form affects physical health, the emotional spirit, and mental stability. The mind motivates and manipulates the activity of the entire body in relationship to the structure. Such harmony develops the possibility of raised levels of consciousness.

Beautifully invisible are the internal features as the player experiences the exercise:

1. Mind is Master:

The mind is perpetually present and vitally engaged during all action—at every second and point of the complex course of the exercise. Its constant presence makes form function physiologically correctly, with psychological ease. Because mind and body work together, the action appears as if spontaneously created with no premeditated plans. The player appreciates the power of mind at all times; without it there is chaos and disharmony.

2. No Effort:

The continually moving figure, gliding on winged feet, presents a picture of effortless activity, giving comfort to the viewing eye and peace to the mind.

2. All Is a Balance of Effort:

The physical forces of effort necessary to activate the process of changes are distributed organically in respect to "need"—some patterns requiring less dynamic tension, others more, each with varying degrees of lightness and strength. The player directs form and the body enacts the effort which is not seen because "tensions" are intrinsic. Effort and form are as balanced as a correctly weighted scale, and so give the look of effortlessness.

3. No Dynamic Changes:

Despite the clearly seen complexities, the combinations of designed patterns, none reveal any emphasis or special accent in the quality of movement manipulation.

3. Constant Variations in Dynamic Tensions:

The muscular system automatically responds to changing formations with a wide range of energetic effort. The player is completely aware of the dynamic action which colors the portrait internally. Perfection of control produces the "even" unwavering aspect.

4. Uniformity:

The many configurations which are amazingly different from each other seem texturally uniform, smoothly and evenly performed with unweighted lightness.

5. The Surface Softness:

The overall impression of the action is one of "softness" in the actual making of the movement because of the fact that no motion shows a trace of tension, and all is maintained steadily and sustained with lightness and ease.

4. Nothing Repeats Itself:

No Form is repeated in exactly the same way because what is considered to be inherent in the Form are the angle of direction it is in, as well as the space-placement—both integral parts of the composition. The player perceives the shades of differences and appreciates the essence of the Forms. What is uniform is the grace and harmony.

5. The Hidden Energy:

The physical body has the power to "call up" just the right amount of force needed for a particular task. This is *intrinsic* effort; for example, clearly legs need more muscle power to function with than do the arms. There is never any need for mind or emotion to demand extra "outside" effort. The mind directs form: the body enacts it, with just the right amount of effort. The visual results of such cooperation makes the action appear to be "soft" (a word that can be misunderstood). Soft is never looseness. Soft is the absence of superfluous tension and contains the hidden energy.

6. Empty-Minded:

A spirit of calmness arising from the unwavering flow of aesthetic images envelopes the spectator, who "mindlessly" becomes restfully relaxed—and who then assumes that the player is empty-minded too.

6. Centered and Concentrated:

Total concentration prevents the mind from wandering off or blanking out. As if impersonal, the quiet face reflects the calmness of the inner self, a calmness that comes from centered awareness of the nature of the intrinsicality of the physical action in the complex structure.

7. Detachment:

With an air of detachment the player seems to be mentally and emotionally oblivious not only of the surroundings, but also of the "self," as if the body were moving along by itself.

7. Deep Involvement:

The player comprehends the substance of T'ai-Chi Ch'uan, appreciates its body-mind harmony, and expects the higher development of self in terms of heart-ease and perceptive insight. The player is totally involved in the process of mind and body.

8. Simplicity:

The entire composition appears as a seamless entity lacking the variable dynamic physical forces necessary for circulating energy to make the body function properly.

8. Multiplicity:

The balanced multiplicity of events: space-time, form, direction, tempo, gravity-force, dynamics—all properly proportioned and therefore in perfect balance—such unity is responsible for the "apparent" simplicity. The means are multiple, the essence simplicity personified.

9. The Ending Mirrors the Beginning

Although the final position at the end of the exercise resembles the one at the starting point, in form and standing posture, the viewer suspects that there is "something" which did not exist at the beginning—an inner sense of effortlessness and repose.

9. At Completion—a New Beginning

The player, when holding the final form impeccably still, experiences the unity of the inner-outer self as being one, undifferentiated. Gradually, a feeling of airy lightness arises, as if free of gravity, heightening awareness and vitality.

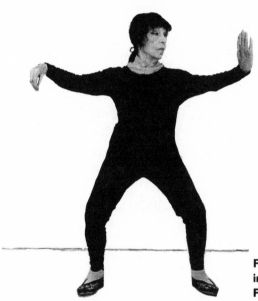

Fig. 6.1 Sophia Delza in Wu style Single Whip Form.

Double Portrait

The images of the portraits are understandably different, but not entirely antithetical. The viewer sees exactly what has been planned by the structure and content of the exercise—as they are being "lived" by the player.

Although obviously the viewer cannot see what lies "beneath the skin," aims and goals are revealed by the external action: the viewer is awakened to a feeling that it is automatically projected through the form.

The player knows what the external effect will inevitably be, since that is the intrinsic nature of the composition and technique—physical, emotional, mental, and philosophical.

What the viewer notes as spontaneity, the player feels is freedom of the spirit. What the viewer sees as effortlessness is a harmonious balance of dynamics for the player. What is detachment for the viewer, the player knows to be centered perceptiveness.

The viewer extracts the appearance from the reality (of the player's action) and appreciates without being able to personally develop from it. The viewer becomes agreeably relaxed from the continually connected patterns. The player is revitalized, alert, and consciously calm.

Despite the fact that the personal "results" differ, the planned external picture, being of the essential technique, and the inner experienced one do make a wholesome whole—a double portrait.

But as noted at the beginning, the presence or reaction of the observer is *never* needed for the player's fulfillment of tranquility.

4. A Refreshing Technique: Action and Thought

At last there is something new in the way of exercising, though it is ancient: an exercise that can be international though it is Chinese, an exercise equally valid for men and women, young and old, artist and artisan. Such is the exercise-art called T'ai-Chi Ch'uan, which I have been teaching to professionals and nonprofessionals. I consider myself fortunate in having been able to study this exercise in China, and happy that as a Westerner, I have been the first to bring this extraordinary and useful technique to the attention of the West.

Can you imagine an exercise which moves you flowingly from Form to Form in slow tempo for not less than 25 minutes, and does not tire you but instead refreshes you? Can you believe that the process of movement is so enjoyable that you emerge from it was a sense of well-being and emotional ease? This ancient Chinese exercise-art is designed to do just that, to activate the body in a total way so that emotional stress disappears, the physical body is strengthened and improved, and the mind is stimulated.

T'ai-Chi Ch'uan uses the body without using it up. Without stirring the heartbeat abnormally, or quickening breathing, it adds energy while building up efficiency; corrects defects; develops endurance without exhausting one. It stimulates mental activity by intricate coordination and through a varied composition, and its smooth, light movements calm the disposition, without which calmness no one could be considered to be truly healthy.

An exercise which claims such benefits effecting mind, body, and the emotions simultaneously, must indeed embody a very special technique, a unique way of moving, and an organization of Forms that differs enormously from the familiar way of the hard-tensed or Western style of exercising.

The following are some of the characteristics of T'ai-Chi Ch'uan from which the reader can get a glimpse of its nature.

1. It is a *slow* exercise. (Hard-tensed style is fast.) The breathing stays natural, the heart steady, the tempo being related to the "good" heartbeat rate. Slowness develops patience, poise, and power.

2. It is called *soft-intrinsic* (which is the opposite of hard-tensed extrinsic). During the process, the muscles are never tensed to their maximum ability. How much effort-tension is used depends entirely upon the demands of the position or movement *itself*. For instance, it is obvious that it requires more energy to stand on one leg than on two. The muscles naturally behave differently in each case. Force is never "inserted" into a movement. "Use one pound to lift one pound." The balance of force with necessity is the "soft" approach, which conserve energy, and awakens one to the proper use of strength.

3. It is *connected* and *flowing*, where each unit, each moment of movement is joined to the next without a visible break. (Hard-Tensed styles accent the finishing of a posture with force.) Calmness and lightness are evoked by such fluidity.

4. It is *continuous*. There is no cessation of movement throughout the entire exercise—like a river it flows on and on. The ability to sustain an even continuity produces stamina and endurance.

5. It is a *complex composition* of multiple themes. (Hard-Tensed style uses short and repeated gestures.) The var-

ied patterns pass from one part of the body to another so that no part is overworked and the mind remains interested.

Good coordination, heightened perceptivity, and improved memory result from being able to execute the varied forms.

6. *Balance,* an essential aspect in dominating the force of gravity, disciplines the movement. Through the control of every nuance, the muscles and joints are subtly strengthened. Proper posture and lightness of movement are inevitable results of good body balance. Balance in its widest sense also contributes to mental and emotional stability.

7. Changes in *dynamics* of light and strong (yin and yang) are in constant alternation. (In hard-tensed style, dynamics are always unvaryingly intense.) Great play in dynamic flow produces flexibility, pliability, resilience, and releases mental tension.

8. It is *circular.* Movements are made in curves, arcs, spirals (in contrast to the angled, hard-edged lines of the hard style.) Moving "in circles" reserves energy, is protective, gives security, and lessens nervousness. It prevents excessive and unneccessary expenditure of force.

9. It is a "from the *mind*" exercise, *the opposite of automatic* and absent-minded behaviour. The mind directs the action and participates in it. This develops concentration, alertness, and personality.

10. *Activity* combined with *stillness* are features which add greatly to control and body awareness. The relationship of these two elements in design promotes restfulness as well as diversity of interest.

11. It is a *long* exercise, a symphonic composition, continuous for 25 minutes. This basic length of time is an essential "ingredient" of T'ai-Chi Ch'uan. It is just long enough

to overcome indisposition and laziness, long enough to impress the body and mind with its many diverse elements, long enough to develop growth in physical strength, patience and persistence, long enough to give every part of the body varied exercise, yet *not* long enough to fatigue.

12. The way of moving is soft, continuous, light, fluid, giving the appearance of effortlessness, yet the body is firm, stable, and strong, the mind alert, active, with consciousness predominating.

What Special Significance Does Such a Technique Have for People in the Performing Arts?

T'ai-Chi Ch'uan is a training preparation for any task (especially for those subject to stage-fright). By doing some of this exercise, the mind is concentrated away from the anxious self and disturbances seem to evaporate. Theatrical life demands a supreme ability to adjust, almost at a moment's notice. To exercise with T'ai-Chi Ch'uan is to become extremely adaptable, calm in emergencies, quick, and pliable. The theater demands endurance, intensive concentration, inventiveness. A serious understanding of one's body movement makes for greater ease and gracefulness in manipulating it for any desired effect. With quickened reflexes, there are speedier responses, an ability to change habits, and to memorize easily. Emotionally there is less self-consciousness and more self-assurance. To work without weariness and with easy proficiency, and especially "to be in harmony" with oneself and one's work are goals everybody desires.

T'ai-Chi Ch'uan can be practiced by each one for different reasons at different times, depending on one's needs. But at all times, it refreshes, lifts the spirits, makes one calmer, and is entirely enjoyable.

5. Perspective on My Experience with the Art of Classical Chinese Theater (Opera)

My first visit backstage in a classical Chinese Theater in Shanghai was a never-to-be-forgotten experience. Had I, at that time, been studying T'ai-Chi Ch'uan, I would certainly have understood and appreciated the special quality of the situation as an actor prepared to make his entrance onto the stage.

I had been in China only two weeks then, but had already attended the theater many times, five hours at each performance, and realized that I was witnessing many times an extraordinary theatrical art. I felt its impact despite my ignorance of play content, costuming, stylization of character roles, music, and language. Even to my novice's eye it was clearly total theater, a synthesis of drama, music, singing, and expressive movement. Subsequently, in my long study of this Classical Chinese Theater art I was to perceive the aesthetic integrity of all its aspects.

Wang Fu-Ying, a most distinguished "action actor" (Wu Sheng) in the Da Wu T'ai Theater in Shanghai, was interested in the fact that I began to study T'ai-Chi Ch'uan with Grandmaster Ma Yueh-Liang. This was after several months of study with him, learning the movement, dance-action, style, and technique of various classical roles.

"And what do you think of T'ai-Chi Ch'uan, and how do you feel about its way of movement?"

"Wang Fu-Ying . . . there seems to be no meeting ground between what you are teaching me so dynamically and the action of this exercise. They differ in rhythm, tempo, dynamics, form, expression, and structure. With you there is dramatic experience and a "giving-out" of feeling. In T'ai-Chi Ch'uan, even as a newcomer, I see that it awakens the power of patience, the development of inner calm, and builds up another kind of energy."

"Absolutely so," said Wang Fu-Ying. "The intrinsic energy each of us in the theater must possess. You will also, eventually, perceive of the exercise's complete harmony. That is not to say that the theater-action does not have harmony, but there is a difference. An actor feels harmony with the character he is playing. T'ai-Chi Ch'uan produces a personal harmony—harmony with one's self."

"Do you yourself play it now?"

"I use it to restore my energy. You know that we have nine performances a week, in a different play each day, and that my roles are very vigorous."

In the ensuing years that followed, as I progressed in each of these arts, we discussed the more subtle qualities of movement and structure, feeling, and expression.

The Classical Chinese theater art is an *extrinsic art*, directed to stir the hearts and minds of an audience, to enlighten and enhance people's knowledge of Chinese history, society, ethics, and art. It is to entertain as well as to educate with dramatic action, song, music, dance, and acrobatics, enriched by the colorful styles of different types of characters.

T'ai-Chi Ch'uan is an *intrinsic art*, directed to stir the heart, mind, and body of the doer, the player of this exercise and to enlighten and enhance the quality of the self. It is never directed outwardly to entertain or inform someone who happens to observe the exercise in action.

The theater actor portrays and projects the situation, thought, and emotion of some other personality, but is never himself personally involved. All techniques are perfected to make him become, for the duration of a play, a character totally different from what he is in his "real life."

In T'ai-Chi Ch'uan one is self-motivated to become a more "advanced" person, to attain emotional stability, physical health, and mental security, to function with a body-mind unity which can be part of one's daily life and work. Inevitably, diligent and conscientious practice leads to the awareness of one's harmonious self-development.

These two arts seem to be worlds apart. Do they, can they, possibly touch at any point of philosophy, ethics, psychology, physiology, or art?

From my long practical experience with the movement-structure of many art styles, I find that the distinctive quality of Chinese movement is a flowing grace, present in every art action style: Dance of the Nationalities, Ancient Palace Dance, Chinese Theater Dance, and the "modern" Ballet, as well as in the exercise-arts of T'ai-Chi Ch'uan, Shao-Lin Ch'uan, Pa Kua Chang Hsing-Yi, and so on. Choreographic unity of space, tempo, dynamics, and form is achieved through this characteristic way of moving, the basic aesthetic element in all action styles.

In T'ai-Chi Ch'uan it is a continuously flowing interconnected form, the integration of coordination, balance (gravitational and structural), and the organic relationship of moving patterns. All symbolically reflect and mirror its aims and goals: calmness, patience, containment, profound perceptivity, and an awakening of higher levels of awareness.

It is in the philosophy of the Chinese classical play that the good must be rewarded and evil punished, that man's personality—his actions and feelings—be the dynamic force and center of interest, that certain virtues be emphasized. Among the latter are respect for family relationships, respect for scholarship, honesty, a sense of humor, and, importantly, a sense of shame. These are to be embedded somewhere in the play's plot. The virtuous hero role is the soul of Chinese theater and has been so from the earliest days of "theater" presentations, as far back as the Chou dynasty, circa 700 B.C.E.

The theater historically reflected a set of values already experienced by the people. Yet it also vividly presented them anew to become ingrained in a "way of life." Whatever the motivation, both attitudes are mutually valid: life creates art, art inspires life.

The art of T'ai-Chi Ch'uan, through its vision and technique, helps man help himself to develop a richer personality and sense of well-being by self-activity on a profound scale. This is clearly different from the "teaching" or intellectualized method to inspire by example of others, as is done in Chinese theater.

From my study of the choreography of the theater's dance action, I appreciated the fact that the composition of each dance is as precisely designed in terms of space, direction, and dynamics as is the structure of T'ai-Chi Ch'uan's forms and transitions—all is a balanced harmony. No personal whim to adjust or rearrange the established patterns is permitted. The organization of "detail" in both arts is impeccably calculated and created to express the organic interconnection of all the elements: space, tempo, direction, and pattern in terms of the physiological changes which make the total body an expressive unity.

In T'ai-Chi Ch'uan, the invisible energy dynamics are "natural" to the activity and are therefore *intrinsic* in quality. In theater action, dynamics convey the emotion and the message dramatically and are *extrinsic* in character.

I now return to my experience backstage to interpret it in the light of my T'ai-Chi Ch'uan knowledge. A backstage atmosphere is always all bustle, with adults and children milling about, chatting gaily without relevance to what is happening so near them on the stage.

Suddenly there was utter silence and all retreated to the farthest corner of the area. An actor had quietly left his dressing room and taken his place about ten feet away from his entrance to the stage. He was calm and stood still and poised, eyes focused toward the stage. He was so concentrated and alert it seemed to me that he might have been as ready to start doing T'ai-Chi Ch'uan as to go on stage.

The unearthly stillness lasted for four or five minutes before the actor stirred, and moving as swiftly and smoothly as if on skates, stopped for a second at the stage entrance, "became" the character he was playing, and leisurely walked onto the stage. At this point, the backstage area once again became alive with chatter and movement as if nothing unusual had occurred.

The actor knows the process of centering and concentration, eliminating all extraneous and irrelevant thoughts. Such a "self" technique is incorporated in the very act of becoming and being a good actor—no matter what the role. Wang Fu-Ying, in my long acquaintance with him, exemplified the naturalness of being calm and contained in teaching and assured in acting, whatever the nature of the roles. It is this "centered" quality that makes the actor a magnetic presence to which the audience deeply responds. However, the actor is concentrated only on his *role*, a personality that is not his own. In T'ai-Chi Ch'uan, the player becomes centered on *himself* alone and is able to retain this concentration in all circumstances, agreeable or not.

From my experience, I do believe that the power of being able to be calm and quiet for theatrical purposes somehow "rubs off" and is absorbed by the private person of the stage actor, even without consciously trying.

To endure night after night, year after year, the arduous life demanded by the theatrical world, the actor undoubtedly possesses, to some degree, the ability to calmly adjust to the facts of everyday living, as he can so easily do in his working life. With T'ai-Chi Ch'uan we are able to find mental balance and equanimity at all times through its harmonious technique and calming spirit.

6. Inherent Qualities: Form, Grace, Stability

Form

After my first lecture-demonstration of T'ai-Chi Ch'uan in New York City (in the late 1950s), a woman came backstage and gleefully said, "What you performed is what I have been doing every day for years."

Needless to say, I was overjoyed. I had just returned from China and as yet had not met anyone who had even the faintest glimmer of the exercise's existence, no less one who actually did it.

I rattled off questions: "When did you learn it and with whom? How long have you been practicing it?"

"Oh no," came the quick answer, "with nobody. I make all the movements up every morning. I just keep stretching and stretching, moving from place to place, and keep going for quite a while."

It was evident to me that she said that she had observed, within the flowing movement, the presence of some forms or patterns which she (mistakenly) took to be personally inspired and spontaneously created at the moment of action, as were her own free-formed, unplanned gestures.

A viewer even on first seeing the complete T'ai-Chi Ch'uan cannot help but be aware that the continuity of the movement connects definitely patterned positions, one to the other.

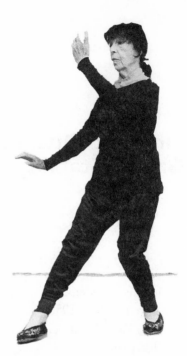

Fig. 6.2 Beginning the Cloud Arms Form

These "positions," inherent in the structure of T'ai-Chi Ch'uan, are the integrated Forms, numbering 108, the building blocks, the scaffolding of the exercise.

Without the clarity of Forms, a continuous stream of activity, with no "stations," so to speak, would become arbitrarily random and would never be a structured part of the composition.

Each Form has a separately distinct meaning, symbolic of the goals of T'ai-Chi Ch'uan.

The transitions, that is, the continuity of flowing patterns, lead to and connect Form to Form, each of which is a momentary point of stillness, wholeness, and completeness, preparing for the beginning of a new transition. Form is the meaning; transition is the process.

Aside from considering a Form as a basis for the application in "self-defense" (that is, combat), a highly developed player aims toward the realization of T'ai-Chi Ch'uan principles through

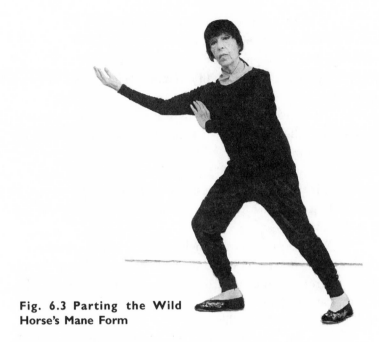

Fig. 6.3 Parting the Wild Horse's Mane Form

the structure of Form, and hopes to attain mental acuity, emotional stability, spiritual balance, as well as physical prowess.

Grace

The grace that is inherent in the action of T'ai-Chi Ch'uan lies in the structural harmony of the complex forms as they are organized to conform to the basic physiological laws of nature.

This grace is not the equivalent of the dancer's grace, nor is it like that of the athlete's.

The dancer imposes on the dance formations personalized expressivity which makes the dance-movement more (or less) fluid, more (or less) emotional, more (or less), continuous—all of which depends on the individual's sensitivity and artistic ability to enhance the dance-forms (which need not be well choreographed!).

The athlete, knowing what the goal to be achieved is, is prepared mentally to adjust body movements so as to accomplish the desired end, with no emotion, no aesthetics.

Regulation of form to express a definite idea creates a harmony that unwittingly becomes a graceful act, but only if the athlete is exact and proficient. The dancer need only contribute to the dance the personal ability to move well in order to appear graceful.

The grace as it appears in T'ai-Chi Ch'uan comes from an entirely different source: it is not personally motivated, nor is it "goal" directed.

The structure itself "possesses" grace through its absolute harmony. It therefore gives, bestows, grace on all who absorb its "laws," as it were, by following the flowing patterns of its profound complexities.

We can say, unhesitatingly, that even the beginning student will be touched by the quality of grace without having done anything, consciously, to acquire it. Why is this so? How is it that an undeveloped student, an "amateur" T'ai-Chi Ch'uan player seems to have bodily grace?

The simple fact is that the organization of T'ai-Chi Ch'uan contains grace; it lies in the very "flesh and bones" (that is, the means and method), and in the essence of its harmony.

All the elements: form, pattern, space-time, dynamics, direction, and the intrinsic energy used in manipulating the action, are so completely in balance that the external harmony of action cannot but be graceful.

The quality of grace is enhanced as the player improves the technical aspect of the integration of the flow of movement and correct form.

Because grace is ingrained in the harmonious structure of T'ai-Chi Ch'uan, the player, in acting consistently with this impeccable exercise-art, has grace "thrust" upon her/him.

Stability

The quality of stability is never strained. It just seems to exist without overt effort in the framework of the total activity.

Correct power in the leg action, with a controlled pelvic area, supports the upper part of the body—torso and head— which therefore can always remain light and "airy."

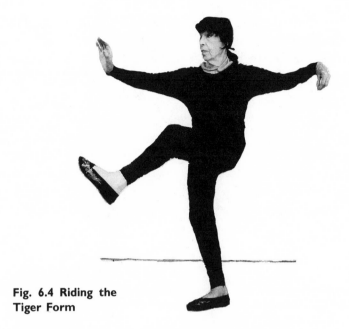

Fig. 6.4 Riding the Tiger Form

Muscular power in various parts of the body is being continually changed dynamically in response both to the demands of formal structure and the shifting positions of leg movements.

No single part of the body is overworked since the yin-yang energy, in varying degrees, travels throughout the system according to the requirements of total balance.

This gravitational stability as seen by an observer is smooth, unwavering action, seemingly without textural variety or dynamic change.

The player experiences the shades of muscular use of strengths and releases, and the constantly interchanging entities of yin and yang. The structure is mathematically regulated to balance inner power and outer form.

Physical activity is not the only element to assure stability.

True stability is more than the ability to withstand gravity. The faultless coordination of the complexities of movements in space and time, and the refinements of bodily changes are the innate ingredients of the "greater" stability, which includes mental and emotional equilibrium.

This is the stability inherent in the philosophy of T'ai-Chi Ch'uan, which is developed with unstrained power, sensitivity, and ease, as the player becomes more physically adept and more perceptive of the full dimensions of the nature of T'ai-Chi Ch'uan.

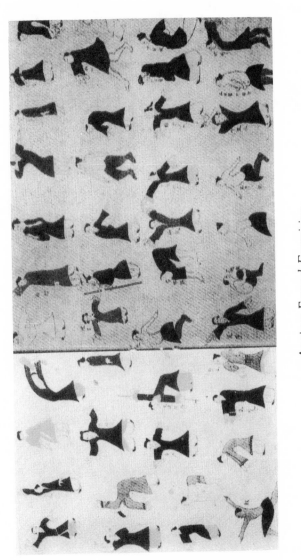

Ancient Formal Exercising

CHAPTER VII

THE STEADY FRAME OF HISTORY

As the eye when focused on a point
Sees it and all the space around
Completely in a circle, so the mind
When centered, is the eye of consciousness
Controlling omnipresent and aware.
Like a magnetbeam, the master-mind
Manipulates with spontaneity
The multifaceted diversities
Of shape and form and space and time.

> Thought and process interwoven
> Motion moving without stopping
> Create the moment harmonized.
> Concentration-integration,
> One with all and all at once,
> Like a shadow's contact with its source.
> Awareness of one's Being, being
> Constant with one's self in one embrace
> > Is triumph of the power of mind and will.   199

The Steady Frame of History

1. Chinese Exercise-Techniques: Kung Fu and T'ai-Chi Ch'uan

One short paragraph in an old guidebook to Beijing made me rise in the cold dawn and hurry down with great excitement to T'ai Miao Park: "The Central Park as well as the T'ai Miao is often frequented in the morning by groups of elderly gentlemen who assemble in a very unaffected way to practice an ancient style of gymnastics."

I had already, in the fall of 1948, after a few weeks in China, seen the subtle movement and the dynamic action of the actor in Classical Chinese theater. I had come across the gay sweetness of the sinuous folk dance from China's far western regions. On the boulevards and in the market places I had been delighted with the fabulous techniques of the traveling street entertainers. Yet the acquaintance with these forms did not prepare me in any way for "the ancient style of gymnastics," so modestly noted in the guidebook.

What I saw was so startling, so interesting from every point of view, that the first impression of the park and the people can never leave my mind. In a vast area, sparsely covered with little islands of grass, but lined with magnificent old cedars whose enormous branches and dense foliage shut out the sky, scores of figures were moving so slowly, so lightly, so continuously that they literally seemed to be floating. Each, in rapt concentration, appeared so weightless, that had one of them risen quietly into the air I doubt that it would have surprised me.

The entire park was alive with these active yet quiet figures. Some, in scattered groups, were led by teachers. Others were practicing individually, in their own ways, no two appearing to do the same thing. Not only were there "elderly gentlemen," as the guidebook said, but also young men and women, too, who were exercising "in a very unaffected way," not in the least affected by each other nor disconcerted by a stranger-onlooker like myself. The Forms being done seemed never to be repeated; the dominating quality was that of movement flowing endlessly, like the perpetual motion of a river. The tempo was slower than slow, as easy and liquid and controlled as the unruffled flow of a slow-motion picture. At first, I felt that I myself had floated into a dream fantasy. But this impression did not last long. Before the dawn had turned to morning and the sun had streaked its way through the thick ancient trees, I experienced the "reality" of the situation—these adults were in no dream trance, but were fully aware of what they were doing. Every day, regularly, before they went to work, they came to the T'ai Miao Park to exercise their minds and bodies in a rich and meaningful way.

I watched an elderly teacher direct his group. He was standing with feet parallel and apart, his knees bent, his back straight. He was illustrating with specific gestures how to "tuck in" the hips, how to grip the ground with the toes, how to direct the knees over the point of the toes (without a sway-back), how properly to curve the outstretched arms while keeping the wrists level. And for a brief moment I thought I was in my own "modern dance" class. But there was a difference, and what a difference it was—for nowhere on the "face" of our Western dance is there to be seen such sustained strength, gentleness, energy without tenseness, such calm or subtle vitality.

I watched the beginners, and others who were beyond the preliminaries, and many others who, it was evident, had been doing the exercises for years. Then I gradually realized that their concentration was not rapt or vacant; that the movements had an extraordinary subtle and fixed pattern; that the people were mentally aware and alert. All of this, I was to learn later, was part of the essence of T'ai-Chi Ch'uan, which is the name of the exercise I was seeing.

My translation of T'ai-Chi Ch'uan is "The Art of Gymnastic Movement," a translation that the following quote from Y. K. Chen's book sheds light on: "To move hands and shoulders, elbows, fists, palms, and fingers; legs, knees, toes, sides of feet and soles . . . so as to form various postures systematically following one another—this is Ch'uan or "boxing." . . . T'ai-Chi means the first principle, or the essence, and embraces the theory of all created things that included both the positive and negative principles—as for instance, activity and inactivity, darkness and light, mobility and rest, etc.—These aspects *supplement* each other; the evolution is infinite. T'ai-Chi Ch'uan therefore embraces the physiological and psychological principles—thus refers to both matter and mind."

The present complete form of T'ai-Chi Ch'uan dates back to 1000 C.E., and is the culmination of centuries of experiment and thought on the subject of exercise for physical, emotional, and intellectual health.

Even from the earliest times in China, a distinction was made between the various forms and uses of body design and body expression: (1) those intended for commemorative and ritual purposes; (2) those intended to stimulate and direct the minds of the audience; (3) those used to stimulate and direct the feelings and the mind of the doer himself. These last were termed medical or health gymnastic movements. Along with arithmetic, music, writing, and dance for ceremony, the dance for health was included in the liberal arts.

It is related that in prehistoric China there had been a great flood which left stagnating waters that infected the atmosphere. Thereupon the ruler Yu (2205 B.C.E.) ordered an organized series of "Great Dances" to be instituted, for, he said, since stagnant waters cause contamination, the same would be true of an inactivated body. By doing exercises to stimulate the circulation of the blood, the body would be refreshed by such activity and therefore would not be subject to disease.

Even these ancient dances dictated by Yu appear to have evolved from inventions of movement for the cure of diseases a thousand years earlier. Though healing with herbs and plants is known to have been practiced even prior to 3000 B.C.E., exercise persisted as an essential, necessary part of curative and preventative medicine. Nearly every medical prescription had its related exercise, but there were infinitely more exercises than medical recipes.

The early Taoists (5th century B.C.E.), withdrawing from society, stressed the observation of nature and natural phenomena as an essential part of their philosophy. This interest led them, among other things, to the study of man's movements in relation to the way he functions physically, emotionally, intellectually, and spiritually. Over the many centuries their followers evolved patterns, postures, rhythmic movements, and breathing exercises which were intended "to develop a clear intellect, ensure good health, and cure complaints."

"Complaints," such as indigestion, asthma, sciatica, tuberculosis, heart ailments, eye and skin diseases (to mention but a few of the "100 illnesses") could be relieved, it was claimed, by specialized postures and exercises done systematically. Remedies for mental and emotional disturbances were given great and equal consideration. Bad or disquieting dreams, grief, langor, "ills of the heart," seemingly baseless fears, indolence, "liking savory things," and insanity (described as the desire to cast off one's clothes and go about naked) were carefully prescribed for. Man's mental, physical, and emotional health was considered in its totality.

In addition to devising ways of curing ailments, an important contribution was made in the techniques to develop the skill in maintaining health and the power to improve it. Gymnastic-exercise, or medical movement, besides being a remedy for disease, was made a branch of education for the healthy person as well.

The term applied to these medical exercises is *Kung-Fu*, meaning "work-man" or "work-done," implying that the man himself does the remedial work for himself; it is not imposed upon him from the outside by doctors or masseurs. The conscious control which he exerts upon himself is the dominating method of "self-improvement." It was believed that "the mechanism is assisted by the postures of the body, by the combined and assorted positions of all the parts. . . . The study of what movements to combine, what to separate, what particular articulations are necessary, results in an enormous number of arrangements, permutations and combinations. To these are added a system of breathing and various positions of lying, standing, sitting, moving (leaps, runs, walks etc.) combining the elements of activity and passivity. . . . Kung-Fu accomplishes the cure of infirmities, restores *harmony* in the body, and therefore man, not disturbed by irregularities, can make himself an instrument of his 'will.' "

In the second century C.E. the surgeon Huat'o, who had experimented with anaesthetics, prescribed systematic exercises which were to be done regularly. He devised "The Frolics of the Five Animals," taking from the individual action of the tiger, bear, deer, monkey, and bird, relevant movement patterns, using jumping, twisting, crawling, swaying, swinging, contractions, and extensions, in such a way as would "promote free circulation of the blood and give the body a feeling of lightness." He recommended that nothing be done to the point of exhaustion, a fundamental principle in the method of T'ai-Chi Ch'uan, which never exhausts, but, on the contrary, produces a feeling of alertness, aliveness, and restfulness, upon completion.

Between the second and the tenth centuries C.E., innumerable gymnastic systems evolved, each created for specific, specialized purposes. A fourth-century boxer wrote a "Canon for Developing the Sinews." Another wrote a treatise on "Deep Breathing as It Relates to Movement." "Lessons for Tensing Movements" became very popular. Exercises in slow and fast tempos were experimented with. Posture-attitudes, allied to a philosophy, became an important part of various cults. All were designed for the improvement of health, both physical and spiritual. None of these forms were ever associated with the "arts" because the different objectives of dance and gymnastic were never lost sight of or confused. Nevertheless, these exercises had a structural form and a designed composition which we have come to associate with "art," and which element contributes vitally to the final objective of experiencing an emotional satisfaction and a sense of equilibrium.

From the sixth century on, the varied and many "National Skills," as they were called, matured and became distinctively organized as to form, philosophy, and purpose. One of these is the Shao Lin style, from the name of the monastery where the Buddhist monk who originated it lived. Shao Lin is an example of the "outer" or hard school of movement as distinguished from the "inner" or soft school. In the "outer" type, muscular action is intense and visible, dynamics are strong and constant, energy is external and forcibly produced. Used more for fighting purposes, it is nevertheless also practiced today as a personal exercise.

All these earlier forms were the seeds from which T'ai-Chi Ch'uan flowered. Branching away from the "outer" style, this vital system is said to embrace the most permanent, profound, and scientific aspects of its predecessors. Its scope was more widely extended to include a technique of heightening perception, increasing the ability to concentrate and coordinate, activating the mind, producing a harmonious equilibrium of movement and thought, and giving a feeling of general all-round well-being.

We are accustomed, in our Western world, to see strength in hardness, vitality in tenseness, and energetic expression in nervousness. The very antithesis is true of "The Art of Gymnastic Movement."

This "inner" or soft school can easily be recognized by the fact that there is no visible exertion in the execution of the movements. The person appears to be completely relaxed, because the designs flow into each other without strain. Actually all the movements are done with a controlled inner force and with "a reserve of energy that is like a bow about to be snapped." "Attention is centered not on the fixed gestures . . . but on the movements changing from one to the other." The continuous movement must pass into and from the positions as smoothly "as a silken thread is pulled out of a cocoon"; they must appear as "solid as water" and have "the balance of a weight." Picturesque similies help to make one understand the qualities in rendering the action: "the form is like that of a bird trying to catch a rabbit"; "the spirit is like a cat waiting to catch a mouse"; "motion should be like refined steel."

There is a continuity in the very slow action of the eyes, hands, feet, body, that produces a feeling of calmness, lightness, and quiet. The doer is, on the one hand, conscious of the interplay of activity and inactivity, of mobility and rest (as "in the flow of a river and stillness of a mountain"); and on the other hand, the structure and techniques are so designed that this consciousness is developed, inevitably, in the process of being done. No matter what the movements—pushing, pressing, lifting, stretching, leglifts, or deep charges, the breath never comes quickly nor is the heartbeat accelerated. This, for the overall purpose of T'ai-Chi Ch'uan, is extremely beneficial.

Vitality is not dissipated as it is in the "hard" type, but is intrinsic and therefore can be stored up. Flexibility and the ability to coordinate quickly cannot be achieved except with alert awareness of every minute action . . . "the mind directs the energy and the energy in turn exercises the body." This is one of the basic principles in the practice of this exercise—that the mind and thoughts are centered on the action.

This brings us to an important point. T'ai-Chi Ch'uan, as with the earlier medical exercises, is for the *doer* only; there need be no audience. The doer is transformed—the doing of it is the being it. This "art" is not intended to affect others. That it is extremely agreeable to watch is due to its integrated formal structure (as complete as a work of "art"), and to the "dance" quality with which the movements are imbued. However, the benefits can be experienced *only* by the doer.

I shall list some of the benefits to be derived from T'ai-Chi Ch'uan as described by my teacher, Ma Yueh Liang, who had already been doing the exercises for thirty years when I began to study with him:

I. The Restoration of Health

Throughout the centuries many cures have been claimed for these exercises. Among the ailments for which this "Art of Gymnastic Movement" is considered a remedy, are anaemia, joint diseases, high blood pressure, gastric disturbances, and tuberculosis. Because T'ai-Chi Ch'uan is done in the open air, because its sustained quiet, slow movements do not stimulate heart action or change one's breathing tempo, because the content of the movement promotes better circulation, and because the totality of the exercise is one of serenity, these curative claims for tuberculosis, especially, should not seem altogether extraordinary to the Westerner whose medical tradition (for T.B.) places such heavy emphasis upon the beneficial effects of rest, sunshine, fresh air, and calm.

2. Emotional Change and "Cultivation of Temperament"

Because of the balance of movements and the method of slowness, lightness, and calmness, it relaxes nervous temperaments, gives one an easy pace and "therefore a good disposition"; it also "rids one of arrogance and conceit."

3. Intellectual and Psychological

With an increase of intrinsic energy, one's interest is heightened: because the techniques involve change and nuance, awareness and mental alertness (T'ai-Chi Ch'uan cannot be done automatically, or while thinking of other things), one becomes more sensitive, and capable of greater understanding. . . . It concentrates the mind. This basic principle of concentration in the execution of the Art of Gymnastic Movement, is a key factor in attaining the final objectives: being calm, sensitive, acquiring energy without tenseness, strength without hardness, vitality without nervousness, and especially experiencing a sense of tranquillity. This is not the tranquillity of inaction, but the tranquillity of the following Chinese definition: "Tranquillity is a kind of vigilant attention. It is when tranquillity is perfect that the human faculties display all their resources, because (then) they are enlightened by reason and sustained by knowledge."

This definition sums up the Chinese point of view, essential in the study of T'ai-Chi Ch'uan. Tranquillity and harmonious functioning of mind and body is directed not toward the obliteration of consciousness, but on the contrary toward heightening it for "useful" purposes.

2. From Youth to Old Age

How often has one heard the remark made by the Chinese or others that T'ai-Chi Ch'uan is an old man's (or woman's) exercise? Photographs in the many Chinese magazines I have seen always show groups of elderly men in T'ai-Chi Ch'uan positions, seemingly moving in unison. Does this make it an old man's exercise, or does it imply that it is an exercise which people, only when older, should learn? Neither is true. T'ai-Chi Ch'uan is an exercise to get older *with*.

By practicing T'ai-Chi Ch'uan for years and years, one will arrive at a good old age with comfort and health. Therefore, T'ai-Chi Ch'uan is a young person's exercise, and my reasoning is simple. It must be learned and studied when one is younger, and it must be practiced and perfected day after day, year after year, in order to reach a ripe old age with stamina and mental agility. Since T'ai-Chi Ch'uan is known as an exercise aiming toward longevity, it must necessarily be started a long time before the great age arrives.

From my teaching experience, I have found that older people (in the United States) who have not exercised when younger have great difficulty in coordinating not only mind with body but also hands and feet. Even if the older person lacks *physical* strength, it does not hamper learning. It is the inability of the mind to be attentive and the body to coordinate with it— as well as the lack of will power to persist—which are the basic reasons for the older person's difficulties in studying.

Since it is the every-changing variety of forms and patterns which are designed to produce balanced health, fine circulation, pliable muscles and joints, it can be seen how important it is to function with that variety of movements so uniquely contained in T'ai-Chi Ch'uan. Therefore, a modicum of the ability to concentrate and coordinate must be present from the very beginning of study. The intricate diversity, stimulates one to become more keenly perceptive and to be ever present. It is the subtle variety which keeps the dynamics of changing energies in moving balance and which brings new and fresh life to the entire system.

It stands to reason, then, that people must start to learn when they are young enough—at that time when they are able to press the mind into attention and to develop the memory more easily, to make the body act in a multitude of ways physiologically, and especially to have the will to persevere with the thought being not on *old* or *any* age, but on physical, emotional, and mental self-development.

How young is young? The twenties are not too young, and certainly the forties and fifties are never too late. But I do believe that the teens are much too young, too early in life experience to be objective and to understand the concept of mental and emotional equilibrium. The teens are the time for exercising with tensed strength, extrinsically, with clearly felt and vigorous physicality. T'ai-Chi Ch'uan requires another kind of mind and muscle intelligence. It demands acute attention, intrinsic and quiet control, and the appreciation and awareness of human potentialities.

People over twenty can give themselves to a new experience willingly and can begin to detect the refinements of a more subtle kind on a more philosophical plane.

Learning at the right time, at a good mental age, one can move through the decades staying young as one's years accumulate. With its structural and philosophical harmony, T'ai-Chi Ch'uan can be considered to be a mature exercise at any age. It is an exercise which all people, as they get older, can continue to do with ease. T'ai-Chi Ch'uan can be designated as "old" if the T'ai-Chi Ch'uanist has lived a long time—long enough to have become wiser while maintaining an active, healthy body and a clear, agile mind. T'ai-Chi Ch'uan is an exercise for men and women of any age "to stay young with."

3. The Art of Wu Shu: Innovations are Changing Traditional Exercises

Wu Shu is an indigenous national exercise-sport the roots of which go back in China's history for thousands of years—to the time when the manipulation of swords, shields, lances, and other instruments of defense and attack were part of commemorative dance and exercise forms.

Throughout the centuries, a great variety of exercise-sports were commonly practiced—archery, wrestling, weightlifting, polo, ball-playing, acrobatics, muscle-building techniques, breathing and movement disciplines—not only, obviously, for physical health but also for the development of a feeling for friendship among those participating.

Wu Shu is the overall name for the different traditional kinds of exercises which have evolved from China's long concern with the health-giving aspects of various types of activity for both body and mind. It includes two schools of exercise which are distinguished by their differing methods, techniques and styles. One is called the soft-intrinsic school; the other, the hard-extrinsic.

The diverse styles of T'ai-Chi Ch'uan, Chang Ch'uan, Hsing I (to name but a few) are examples of the soft-intrinsic school, the techniques of which are unique in the world history of exercise. This school is characterized by the fact that there are no signs of visible exertion or expenditure of energy while executing the forms, which are made to flow continuously one into the other without strain and without any stopping in the long structure. The harmonious balance of forces and inner dynamics is a "soft" appearance outwardly, whereas the inner feeling is strong, firm, and secure. Since the tempo is slow and no part of the body is overworked, the heartbeat and the breathing are never speeded up.

Hundreds of Styles

In the hard-extrinsic school of Wu Shu are included hundreds of styles of traditional exercises, their techniques being the very opposite of what is described above. All the Kung Fu exercises are fast-moving, with visible projections of force and dynamics; the routines are relatively short. Leg and footwork are extremely speedy; leaping, jumping, bounding, somersaulting, kicking, and acrobatic gyrations are all used in combination in this extrinsic Wu Shu. Intricately designed manipulation of single- and double-edged swords, spears, staffs, and the like, is intrinsically part of this style of activity—as well as the use of the "empty" hand.

At one of the Spare-Time Schools in Beijing we were presented with a continuous performance (more than two hours long) of Wu Shu techniques done by girls and boys who dazzled us with their technical prowess, grace, and coordinated skills. We were shown the basic practice techniques—the designed structures for arms and wrists, body, head-eyes, and foot-leg work; combinations of attitudes, stances, postures, with units of movements; fencing with broadswords in twos and threes; solo sword play; group action in complicated routines requiring leaps, arabesques, floor patterns, air twisting-turns—all in rhythmic routines perfectly balanced and timed. The dexterous students, so marvelously disciplined, maintained their quiet and composed manner throughout these extraordinary and physically difficult techniques.

This fast-moving Wu Shu is taught at the Spare-Time Schools which students attend after their regular school day to learn the athletic sports they prefer—besides the art of Wu Shu, basketball, table tennis, volleyball, skating, swimming, and various types of acrobatic gymnastics are taught. These schools promote culture and build up health—an all-round development, morally, physically, and intellectually. Between the ages of 7 and 16 the students go for either three-month or six-month sessions after which the best students help with the gymnastic training in their schools. Some continue their disciplines and enter national competitions. In the particular school we visited there are three enormous outdoor playgrounds and immense indoor gymnasiums. There are 160 full-time workers and staff members; the teachers are all experienced professionals. All schools and equipment are free.

A Period of Innovating

Many innovations are being made in the field of Wu Shu. In the People's Republic of China today, the fast Wu Shu is being made creatively more complex, whereas the slow Wu Shu—T'ai-Chi Ch'uan—has been simplified. Originally (for at least 100 years) T'ai-Chi Ch'uan was twenty-two to twenty-five minutes long and continuously performed without any break; the ability to do this assured one of developing stamina, endurance, concentration, and patience (since time is of the essence!). Today the popular version is 6–8 minutes long, made so to meet the needs of the great mass of people. Although this shortened version reduces the number of subtle movements for better body action and narrows the extent to which one builds up endurance, concentration, and control, nevertheless, the requirements for perfection in rendering the harmonious movements and forms are definitely strict and excellent results can be felt.

The fast Wu Shu, on the other hand, is being extended and expanded creatively to increase the agility, speed, skill, and dexterity of the performer. Not chained to the simple forms of the past, the routines are being lengthened and elaborated (for example, increased from 30 to 70 forms), not only for greater stamina but also for quicker reflex action, deeper perception, an ability to adapt to changing situations, and especially for more strategic subtlety. Floor patterns depart from the straight line and are intricately interwoven in curves and zigzags, which coordinate with the more intricately arranged footwork and weapon play—in group or solo action.

The possibilities for the development of this technique are seemingly without creative end. In the style and art of Wu Shu the way is wide open to "bring forth the new" from this ancient and technically extraordinary exercise-sport.

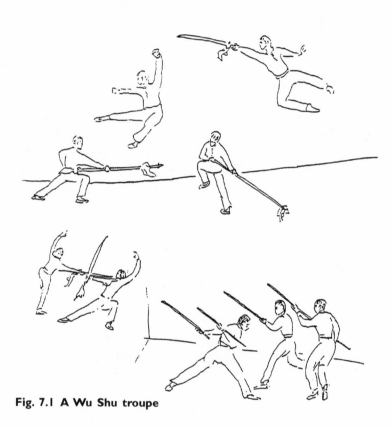

Fig. 7.1 A Wu Shu troupe

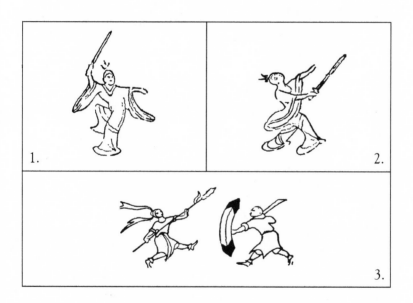

Old Forms Actual Today

4. Chinese Exercise-Arts from Antiquity to the Present

In B.C. twenty-two-o-five
(as I've heard tell)
Chinese Emperor Yu knew how
to help his people stay alive
and well, with movements he
created—rhythmic dance (now
as then called "Great"), to animate
the body-system's circulation
in order to prevent disease-
bearing stagnation; Yu believed
this to be so, based on his
scientific observation,
four thousand years ago.

> Down the ages, at various
> stages of China's long history,
> a wealth of constructive ways
> were devised to stabilize health
> and the act of living
> mindfully; from contemplation
> of the world of nature,
> to imitate, for ease and
> flexibility, the way of

birds and beasts (at least a few);
with due consideration of
the heavenly way, to imitate
and emulate the constant
ebb and flow of rhythmic energy
for long-time stimulation of
wellness and longevity.
Century after century
increasing perceptivity
gave inspiration for body-
movement combinations requiring
subtle manipulation and complexity:
engaging space-time-place
significantly, stabilizing
mind with gesture patterns
organized with structured
unity of form and substance
gradually making progress to a
higher level of consciousness.
Basic organic physicality
involved harmoniously
with mental regulation
laid a firm foundation
for an integrated exercise
utilizing intricate technique
for body-mind awareness—which
reached a peak in the masterly
choreography of T'ai-Chi Ch'uan,
expressing physicological philosophy
of action and tranquility:
T'ai-Chi Ch'uan, the exercise-art for everyone.
This presently popular exercise
(a few hundred years extant),

in some coming century
will I surmise attain
a *newly* structured frame,
retaining—as has been true
since 2205 B.C.—
the natural content of
Nature's intrinsicality:
The spine and core, the concept-
thought that every woman, every man
can begin to cultivate with
conscious discipline a mindful,
healthy, long life-span.
>Yet *another* Ch'uan dimension, enriched
>in Form and Activity, will emerge
>in an evolutionary way,
>urged on by mature comprehension
>and keen sensitivity to man's
>potential for self-harmony.
And what will that be?
Can you perhaps, please tell me!

CHAPTER VIII

CAUTIONARY COMMENTS

T'ai-Chi Ch'uan is *lived* not "played at"
In the process of each doing,
Unifying meaning-movement,
Logic-symbol, structure-substance,
Fact and image interactions,
Real and magic interweavings,
Dynamic and organic body ease
With easy breath and quiet heart, comes
From cultivation of the natural.

> Creating calm, longevity,
> Keener insight and awareness
> To society and self, T'ai-Chi Ch'uan
> Completes a circle (cycle), expressed
> In matter (form) and motion (breath)
> With time not counting time (as space)
> Returning to the point where it began,
> With consciousness enlivened,
> > Finding, in the end, a new beginning.

Cautionary Comments

I. On the Necessity of Never Omitting *Ch'uan* in T'ai-Chi Ch'uan

When I am asked on the telephone whether this is the *T'ai-Chi* School, I say, No, this is the T'ai-Chi *Ch'uan* School, and the caller is flabbergasted.

For many years, and I could say decades, I have been trying to correct people who talk about *T'ai-Chi* as if it were the exercise. Even those who are studying rarely know that it is the *ch'uan* which is the exercise and that T'ai-Chi is the *way*. I try to explain that the *ch'uan* (the exercise) is modified by T'ai-Chi which is its philosophy and which incorporates the principles of balanced harmony: the T'ai-Chi way by which the *ch'uan* is formed.

By way of simple explanation, I suggest to various people that they think of the use of the word *modern* in our world today. If I were to say I study *modern* the obvious question would be—modern what?—painting, dance, science, history, philosophy, economics? As far as the Chinese are concerned, studying *T'ai-Chi* means *little*, unless amplified by an "idea."

There are many *ch'uan* in China—hundreds of forms, styles, types of exercises. The two great systematic divisions are (1) *ch'uan* which are intrinsic (called Nei-Chia) and (2) those which are extrinsic (Wai-Chia). There are innumerable extrinsic *ch'uan* and only one *T'ai-Chi* Ch'uan (intrinsic). This system has a few variations as distinguished by different masters' creative viewpoints: as the Chen, Yang, Wu, Sun, Ho (and perhaps other) styles.

I do appreciate the fact that T'ai-Chi is a short-cut of speech—but sadly it is also a short-cut of thought and knowledge. I say this quite freely since I have read many books and articles which express the authors' understanding of T'ai-Chi Ch'uan profoundly. But, sadly again, these writers speak of *T'ai-Chi* as if they didn't know anything about the existence of Ch'uan and did not suspect that T'ai-Chi is *not* the exercise (otherwise they certainly could have explained the use of the "short-cut"). In Chinese publications, *taijiquan* (T'ai-Chi Ch'uan) is *never* shortened.

This comment is directed to those who, though conscientious, may have been misled, and to those who understand how easily the essence of an idea can be lost through ignorance or carelessness—especially when one is seriously involved in doing and learning this extraordinary, harmonious exercise called T'ai-Chi Ch'uan.

2. Is T'ai-Chi Ch'uan "Martial"?

In many years of study in Shanghai, I never heard the word "martial" used—neither in English nor in Chinese—in connection with T'ai-Chi Ch'uan; nor had I read, in the books translated for me, any ideas implying a martial (that is, military) spirit embedded in this exercise.

Grandmaster Ma Yueh-Liang made it clear to me while I was studying with him that T'ai-Chi Ch'uan was a "from the mind" exercise for total self-development: a discipline which activated the body and mind harmoniously, and which, at the same time, increased the possibility of attaining a higher level of awareness and perceptivity.

The obvious first line of "self-defense" is to prevent weakness and ill health. Also incorporated in its method and structured patterns, forms, and transitions, are physical and technical ways of movement enabling one to defend oneself against an aggressor.

This exercise does not include, even for a fleeting second, the concept of acting aggressively, that is, martially, which reflects military (army) training. And here I come to the point: The concept and use of the word "martial" with T'ai-Chi Ch'uan is relatively recent. Especially emphasized in the West, "martial" is added, indiscriminately, to any Eastern exercise activity which demands physical prowess.

When T'ai-Chi Ch'uan is included under the heading of martial arts, it misdirects (and abuses) the essence of its peaceful nonaggressive qualities, and also belittles its self-defense character.

Somewhere and at sometime the word "martial" was substituted for the idea of discipline in T'ai-Chi Ch'uan, according to Ralph C. Croizier in his book *Traditional Medicine in Modern China*.

I paraphrase him freely: When the authorities of the Imperial troops observed that the soldiers had become lazy, enervated, and weak-willed because of inactivity between war campaigns, they devised a rigid system of exercises to maintain and increase basic bodily strength and stamina.

The military routines were mandatory, to be done systematically and regularly, as a martial (i.e., military) discipline for all Imperial troops.

Because T'ai-Chi Ch'uan is an exercise to be practiced every day, with strict adherence to form and content, it was said to have "discipline" like that of the army's—but only in the sense that it required unremitting diligence, serious applications, and daily practice.

When "martial" took the place of the word "discipline" as a descriptive term for the military, it is thought that T'ai-Chi Ch'uan acquired the word "martial," displacing "a discipline like that of."

The content, techniques, and goals of each were ignored in the designation of that term.

I know that the word "martial" (art) is in use in China at present, but I believe it is being done so in imitation of the American (and English) way, which lumps all Eastern exercise forms under the martial arts.

Under Wu Shu, the art of physical exercise in China, there are two separate disciplines—one Shaolin Ch'uan, which is described as *Wai* (extrinsic), and the other T'ai-Chi Ch'uan, which is described as *Nei* (intrinsic).

Historically, T'ai-Chi Ch'uan is a body-mind discipline based on the harmony of body-action, not a martial (i.e., military) art.

Army exercise routines in no way resemble any aspect of T'ai-Chi Ch'uan forms—not in tempo, structure, yin-yang dynamics, harmonious structure, not in the intrinsic (no tenseness) nature of movement, and certainly not in goals.

T'ai-Chi Ch'uan can self-defend, but it does not "offend."

This story may be pertinent. A monk entered an inn in a village somewhere in China. A group of hoodlums (bandits) were having a gay time. One of them thought it would be a pleasant diversion to attack the monk.

He approached the weak-looking monk, who facing the bandit, kept walking backwards slowly as if in fear.

When the monk neared the back wall, the bandit made a speedy lunge at him just as quickly the monk moved out of his path to one side. The bandit crashed with full force against the wall. The monk quietly walked out of the inn.

That is self-defense (and not martial)!

3. On Martial Art "Experts"

I would like to make some cautionary comments on the practice of T'ai-Chi Ch'uan by exponents of martial self-defense action.

It can be assumed that all the martial-art-defense exponents have been disciplined by the philosophy, technique, and spirit of T'ai-Chi Ch'uan (no matter which style).

T'ai-Chi Ch'uan embodies qualities and goals that can inspire one to "move" or to follow different roads, on the physical, emotional-mental, or spiritual level; or to move "outward" to apply certain essentials to the self-defense aspect of the martial (military) art.

Over these past years, many men (no women) have visited me at my studio to show me, privately, their renditions of T'ai-Chi Ch'uan, which had inspired them to study self-defense action. All of these people considered themselves to be experts.

In all cases (with one exception), what I witnessed was T'ai-Chi Ch'uan imbued with qualities which are extraneous to it: assertiveness, speed, combativeness, super energy, looseness of structure (Forms not completed, etc.), and a confident, complacent feeling of self-satisfaction.

In other words, the effect was indistinguishable from a "practice" of self-defense, vigorous and extrinsic. The practitioners had forgotten the "steps" by which they had ascended (that is, T'ai-Chi Ch'uan) to progress to another type of movement and spirit necessary for defensive action. They had lost (perhaps) the spirit of T'ai-Chi Ch'uan; the harmony of slow tempo, clarity, continuity, balanced yin-yang dynamics, multiplicity of subtle form-patterns, intrinsicality, lightness, and centeredness, all of which, used correctly, can give insight, prowess, and power to other kinds of action (Kung Fu); qualities which give speed, alacrity, flexibility, perceptiveness, and instantaneous reflexes.

I am simply writing this as a cautionary note (if I may be so presumptuous). But please note that I have witnessed and been with the great Grandmaster Ma Yueh-Liang in Shanghai (my teacher) when he performed T'ai-Chi Ch'uan with intrinsic ease, stamina, and spirit, even though he is almost beyond compare in the arts of self-defense and is a master of Ch'i Kung healing. The video-film recently shown on PBS—"Mystery of Ch'i"—reveals the utter quietness of his action in T'ai-Chi Ch'uan.

Mr. Chen Kung in his two-volume book, *The Composite Study of T'ai-Chi Ch'uan and the Related Ch'uan Shu (Motion Arts)*, firmly stresses that one must practice and persevere with T'ai-Chi Ch'uan at all times—a requirement even for expert self-defense people.

4. A Letter on the Subject of Music

I feel that I must comment on the common statement that music can be used to create coordination of body and mind in T'ai-Chi Ch'uan.

If T'ai-Chi Ch'uan itself does not do this, then T'ai-Chi Ch'uan as a "from the mind" exercise is worth nothing because then it is lacking the very principle which it claims for its existence—putting body and mind into harmony *without* outside assistance.

T'ai-Chi Ch'uan exists for itself, in itself, and by itself through the very complex nature of its own physical, mental, emotional world. Music is extraneous to the essence of T'ai-Chi Ch'uan. It is a distraction, a crutch, to woo and reduce the student into thinking that calmness is being attained. It is a deception to make T'ai-Chi Ch'uan palatable by romanticizing the exercise.

Actually, music prevents the doer from concentrating on the harmonious relationship of form and self, of being "aware" and developing insight and conscious tranquillity.

Instead of "listening" to *oneself*, with *music* one leans on the outside sound, which undermines the essential spirit of T'ai-Chi Ch'uan. Away with the notion that sound must bombard the ears.

Also, I wish to comment on recent Wu Shu performances in New York City in respect to the *music* problem. For theatrical purposes, the directors (American?) added trivial music to some of the Wu Shu numbers. By tradition, all *ch'uan* (exercises)—Pa Kua, Hsing Yi, Shao Lin, and so on—are done without sound since the inner aspect of each of the systems is integrated with itself.

Music was used to fill the audiences' ears. The performers completely ignored the music. This was obvious to me since the music *never* ended with the particular number and had to be stopped in the middle of a phrase—like circus music—when the number was concluded.

Sadly, the Chen style of T'ai-Chi Ch'uan was performed almost literally with melodic music, making the movements and structure romantic, overdressed, sentimental, and ornate. I hasten to add that the performers were excellent.

I repeat . . . *away* with music when it does not belong to the *action*.

In China (disregarding the exhibition!) there is *no* sound accompaniment to *any ch'uan* (exercise), past or present.

5. T'ai-Chi Ch'uan Is Not Moving Meditation

The word *meditation* has caught on like wildfire in the United States. It is exploited in many fields of endeavor and is commonly used for "stopping and thinking a bit." Even elementary teachers tell their pupils to "meditate"—meaning, "Don't fidget, sit still, don't bother me, keep quiet." That would be all well and good if there were some guidance as to how to behave in that way.

Meditation is too serious a discipline to be treated trivially and incorrectly, especially by those who do T'ai-Chi Ch'uan. This is my point—it is utterly false to term this exercise, which demands constant mental attention, "meditation in movement," as is being done today by some.

T'ai-Chi Ch'uan, through its harmonious structure, aims at and succeeds in making one centered, calm, serene, and quiet. Do not confuse it with the act of meditation—the methodical process of each being antithetical. T'ai-Chi Ch'uan is a body exercise with mind present and alert. Meditation is no movement and no-mind, the suspension of mind.

T'ai-Chi Ch'uan is movement and form in changing aspects of unified *action* during which one is on one's *feet* all the time and meditation is the "sitting quiet" technique. To move in T'ai-Chi Ch'uan is to be *with* the action, sharpening mind and perception, finding and achieving the unity in multiplicities.

Therefore, mind disciplines the body and the body disciplines the mind in the harmony of differentiated activity.

T'ai-Chi Ch'uan is mind-controlled movement. Meditation is no movement and no-mind, or mind emptying. Yet we must emphasize that T'ai-Chi Ch'uan puts one into a state of Being (a frame of heart-mind) which makes one more easily receptive to the meditation process.

Y. K. Chen in his book on T'ai-Chi Ch'uan says that T'ai-Chi Ch'uan is preparation for meditation. Why and how it is preparation can easily be understood—it eliminates random and irrelevant thoughts. It "eases" emotionality so that concentrating is made less difficult.

Nancy Wilson Ross in her book on Buddhism says that the monks, after *sitting* in meditation from seven to eight hours, are told to walk around and *continue* their meditation. This is *not* meditation in movement. They are continuing what they have done for many hours, while loosening their joints, restoring circulation, and stretching their muscles. Walking takes no effort mentally. It is a mechanical, instinctive act, a natural, simple process having *no* coordinative difficulties. Therefore, meditation can go on without thinking of what the body is doing.

Mistakenly, this, to Western minds, became meditation in movement—an impossibility in T'ai-Chi Ch'uan with its complexities of form and action and its dynamic power of yin and yang.

One moment of no-mind while practicing T'ai-Chi Ch'uan and the moving person would flounder in a sea of mistakes. The body must be with the mind and the mind with the body—in harmony and attentive at all times to each other.

6. On the Spirit in Teaching

When teaching T'ai-Chi Ch'uan, the instructor must be aware that it is almost impossible to neglect its inner meaning, since each one of its aspects—physical, mental, and emotional—is totally enmeshed with the other. It is impossible to treat these elements as if they appeared in layers, one on top of the others, or each exclusive of the others.

The new student, although bound to the physical process at first, can be made to feel, by correct integrated teaching, that the mind-body-feeling relationship is "one"; that the feeling of ease comes from such interaction as well as from the nature of T'ai-Chi Ch'uan's structure itself—its fluid continuity and diversified material which entices the mind. The student must also be made aware that only through *correct* physiological technique can the structure and the "human" body achieve a unity— a harmonious wholeness.

The teaching process has to be rich in idea (and references); discerning as to the range of information given at one time; astute as to when to bring out the subtle and abstract necessities. Teaching creatively, not mechanically, the teacher knows how to keep in step with the student's ability to absorb and integrate concepts which may lead to higher levels of awareness.

The Western student needs the "word" to explain what the eye alone cannot perceive—the accurate position of space and structure large and small (so easily understood in China).

The kinesthetic sense and sensation is gradually felt with the clarifying help of analyzing exactly what and where as well as how. A gesture is made: a wave, an arc, a parabola become "concrete"; the dynamics of weight and release, and of tempo and space, are recognized "bodily" if and when they are first "scientifically" explained. But the teacher must know how to make the student adapt to a "reality" of body movement without interfering with or neglecting the "heart-felt" experience of being patient, calm, and at ease—during the long (and welcome) practice of learning.

The teacher is indeed *responsible*, but if inspired to teach, can bear this burden easily.

7. Street Scene at Dawn: People Exercising

For the visitor in China, to get up early is more than its own reward. My stroll between 5 and 7 a.m. on Chang An Avenue in Beijing would have been (had I not known it already from past experience) an introduction to the fact that the Chinese people believe that exercise contributes to good health and well-being.

What I saw in the cool dawn was taking place all over China, at least in the big cities which I visited.

Parks, streets, squares, open areas under trees, on curbs and sidewalks—all were astir with figures concentrating on various kinds of exercises. Everywhere one looked, people of all ages were seriously engaged in quiet movement. Some were organized in groups; some were moving individually. Scores were being taught a regulated system by a teacher, while many were manipulating their bodies in personal patterns of movements.

Generally speaking, the activities I observed were of two kinds. The style which hundreds of people were intently doing or learning and which clearly dominated the scene was *T'ai-Chi Ch'uan*. This traditional exercise, going back hundreds of years, is of the soft-intrinsic school in which the designed forms are performed without stopping in a continuous and flowing manner. The patterns are so intricately varied as to activate the entire body in a total way which insures physical, emotional, and mental well-being. The other type was what I designate as gymnastic-calisthenic, in which simple movements are repeated without variation.

The first person I saw one early morning in Beijing was an elderly man facing a tall hedge and evidently breathing in its dewy freshness. At his side was a little girl imitating her grandfather's actions. Standing simply, with arms loosely hanging at his sides, the man was slowly circling his head, first to one side many times, then changing to the other. After that he placed his hands on his hips and pushed his body from side to side. He then took a wide stride and loosely bent his torso right and left. Finally he bent one knee and straightened the other alternately. He did this about forty times, maintaining a leisurely tempo and a regular rhythm throughout.

From where I stood I could see others going through their routines—a very old woman, poised at the curb, was swinging her arms forward and back, bending and unbending her wrists, giving her hands special attention. In the distance was the silhouette of a man who had one foot placed high up on the trunk of a tree, using it as we do a ballet-barre; he lowered his torso to touch the foot of the standing leg, lifting and bending repeatedly. Holding hands, a couple paced to and fro under the trees, taking large steps with knees raised exaggeratedly high; they took twenty steps forward and retraced their path. On cold mornings many went through their exercises heavily clothed and wearing gloves, which did not impede their movements or diminish their serene concentration, or even interfere with their easy and light movement. In several weeks of observation I never saw anyone move fiercely, violently, or speedily—differing in this respect from our Western calisthenics, which are usually tense and fast.

But what really commanded attention and filled the landscape in every city at dawn, were the immense numbers of people practicing T'ai-Chi Ch'uan.

A great contrast to the slow-moving T'ai-Chi Ch'uan practitioners were the vigorous young boys being taught the fast, extrinsic style of Kung Fu. On another day I saw a large group

of boys being trained to run swiftly—trotting their way in a
wavelike path, in and out of a line of regularly spaced trees, or
dashing up and down the steps of a concert hall, increasing their
speed on each repetition.

Exercise is prevalent at every stage of a person's development in the People's Republic of China, from early childhood
to a mature age. Nursery children are given various kinds of
dances; school-age children engage in gymnastics, acrobatics, and
dance. Sports of all kinds are popular. There are Spare-Time
Schools where techniques of all kinds are taught, from sport
activity and Western gymnastics to the traditional Wu Shu, an
elaborate technique for body development through structural
forms which use such properties as swords and lances. And there
are the dance schools by the hundreds for amateurs, and professional schools for the professionals-to-be.

For those who, self-directed, wish to exercise freely, and
for those who like to practice on their own, the early morning
is the most suitable time, from the point of view of fresh air and
leisure, to put oneself into a healthy physical state and an agreeable frame of mind before attending to the work of the day.
Exercising in the open air at dawn is truly a people's movement
for health and longevity in China today, as it has been in
the past.

8. On the Abridged Version of T'ai-Chi Ch'uan

I do not wish to offend those who so sincerely practice the short-ened version of T'ai-Chi Ch'uan, who, of course, benefit greatly from its slow tempo, fluidity, and basic variety of movements. However, I wish to make clear and explain in what respects it falls short of the intrinsic long style of T'ai-Chi Ch'uan, where struc-ture and "time" meet on physical, emotional, mental, and aes-thetic levels simultaneously.

T'ai-Chi Ch'uan, as it is practiced today in its 25–30-minute length, is somewhat shorter than it was originally in the twelfth–thirteenth centuries. Nevertheless, at its present length, its composite technique can fulfill the aims and goals designed for man's longevity: fine physical health, stable disposition and mental alertness. We must never forget the T'ai-Chi Ch'uan is called "from the mind" exercise.

The very short version of T'ai-Chi Ch'uan was devised in China. Not only because it is a mere 6–8 minutes long but also because of the arbitrariness of the structured sequences, it cannot and will never help one to achieve the hoped-for long-term goals—physically, emotionally, or mentally.

It is argued that most people today: (1) do not have pa-tience to do lengthy forms; (2) cannot concentrate beyond a certain minimal point; (3) have no "time" to exercise; (4) are too nervous to stay at one thing for any length of time; (5) are not interested in the "mind" aspect; (6) are too restless to persevere.

These are the reasons for which T'ai-Chi Ch'uan has been so drastically shortened, the very reasons it should *not* have been, since the essential purpose of this exercise is to develop a person in all of those aspects harmoniously: in patience, calmness, concentration, ease, mental agility, and physical prowess.

The shortened version of T'ai-Chi Ch'uan can never develop the following:

1. Good physical health: The immense variety of movements in the longer style, the diverse forms and placements with their multiple dynamic changes, reach every part of the body internally and externally in proper harmonious order and balance. Obviously, with fewer movements to perform, the body can only be partially activated, and then not very subtly.

2. Concentration and mental stimulation: A long exercise requires that one remember many more intricate movements and variations, to perfect and integrate them. With less to think about and to do, as in the short form, these metal and physical aspects do not progress to higher stages of development.

3. Coordination: Elaborate and complex coordinative "problems" keep the mind active and make the body more versatile and adept. The higher the level is for the demands of physical activity, the greater and more subtle is the balance of body and mind. The shortened exercise requires less need for skillful coordination, thereby keeping the mind from being fully occupied.

4. Patience: The accumulation of complex activity, slow and ceaseless, in a continually changing structure, develops an inner sense of calm and patience when one gives oneself to a "lengthy" process. Patience begets patience. It is necessary to go beyond ordinary interest and attention to acquire effective understanding of one's emotional state and accumulate, so to speak, the spirit of

patience—which can be naturally applied to and ever
present in one's daily work.

5. Profound awareness and perception: Deeply necessary for
   mental agility, this is being advanced constantly as the
   action of form-dynamics-structure evolves and makes
   "impression" on the consciousness. In a short exercise,
   since the forms are few and the connectives simple, this
   cannot happen. Greater power in understanding the self
   ensues from the intricacies and subtleties as they are
   organized in multifaceted and complicated relationships.

6. Structure: The composition of the entire exercise must
   not be broken up because the nature of the changes are
   intrinsic and physiologically correct according to nature's
   laws, balanced as they are by shape, dynamics, direction,
   and space, as well as structure, all of which are function-
   ally aesthetic as well. There is unity in theme and variations; unity in the use of the body's forces; unity in outer
   aspects of the eight directions; unity in repetitions and
   changes—all of which contribute to calmness and contentment. How can one expect an arbitrarily juxtaposed,
   simplified series of movements which have no intrinsic
   logic to accomplish this? The structural harmony which
   affects the spirit and mind has been destroyed in the
   rearranged short version.

7. Heartbeat and breath: To sustain an even breathing rate
   with a regular heartbeat while performing the complete
   T'ai-Chi Ch'uan indicates that the technique is correct
   and that the person is well-developed. To do the same
   action for a few minutes means little or nothing at all in
   respect to a reserve of energy and the development of
   intrinsic strength. To be able to sustain the tempo of
   constantly changing movements with minimum effort is
   proof of stamina and correct action (actually in the long
   style the pulse will become slightly slower).

8. Endurance: Power and endurance are developed only by time, effort, and perseverance. The ability to perform the exercise for a longer and longer period with the correct degree of slowness, continuity, fluidity, clarity, and physical ease, proves that there is real and easy strength, with inner and outer control of physical, mental, and emotional balance. With time and practice, all can acquire the power of endurance. Short and slow exercise cannot possibly produce power to this same degree. The short exercise does not give the body-time enough to warm up, from which point (in long style, after 8 or 10 minutes) the body is lubricated and made more pliable by the gradual increase of elasticity in the muscles and joints. The short exercise stops at this important point—6–8 minutes, when the slow action just begins to warm up the body.

Any exercise has its virtues. The very fact of doing something extra with body movement is advantageous—but to what degree and to what end? The heart of the matter in the long T'ai-Chi Ch'uan is that it is harmoniously complete at every level for the accomplishments of its basic principles for body-mind-spirit.

If the mental aims are not too high and the satisfaction of doing a few forms is agreeable, then the short version is certainly sufficient. But it is necessary to note that the short series falls far short of the long-term goals necessary for the total health of the player—values so uniquely and masterfully conceived in the profound and long T'ai-Chi Ch'uan.

9. On Traditional Clothing for Practice

It would not be wise to disturb the new student with too many orders as to what to wear, except for the basic necessities. When the student has experienced some aspects of the exercise, and begins to appreciate what the ultimate benefits will be—on a physical, "medical" level—then it is time for them to be told what requirements have existed traditionally and why it is best to follow them.

To put it directly, before I describe the clothes, what is taken as a basic consideration is how the skin functions during exercising, which is as important as the way one's muscles and joints behave.

The act of perspiring is taken for granted, but the "rate" of its increasing activity is also an essential part of the philosophy of health and endurance in T'ai-Chi Ch'uan movement.

I was informed by Grandmaster Ma Yueh-Liang, when I was studying in Shanghai, that because the method is basically directed toward health and longevity, by means of intrinsic slow action, with heartbeat and breathing regularity, the acceleration of perspiration must be gradual. After about 8–10 consecutive minutes, the body warms up and shows some perspiration; and eventually for the continuing 20 minutes or so, the entire body is suffused with warmth.

Not only is perspiring important—but also the way it evaporates.

And so I come to the point of what to wear: long-sleeved top (shirt), long pants or slacks, torso, of course, is covered to neck. Clothing must be loose to permit the skin to breathe (no tight leotards); material, obviously light-weight depending on the weather, indoors or out. Slippers—never bare feet—light-weight with flat soles. Soles of feet are very sensitive to the cold or heat, and slippers avoid friction when moving heels or toes.

Many students wear short, T-shirts, and so on. The arms and legs are cooled more quickly than the torso and trunk. So the advantage of an evenly "tempered" body is lost.

Our skin-organ's reaction is utterly vital to health. The proper clothing aids its functioning in respect to the demands of the T'ai-Chi Ch'uan organization of patterns and forms.

When one is truly a T'ai-Chi Ch'uan player, knowledge-able and developing on higher levels physically and mentally, full dress will almost be automatic and the body will then naturally do its own work in terms of proper circulation. T'ai-Chi Ch'uan is performed for the sake of the player—and not for *show*.

CHAPTER IX

LIGHT VERSE ON *SERIOUS* *THEMES*

An Art of Exercise,
Formed to flow in silence,
   Has an eloquence
That radiates the essence of
   Calmness, ease and patience, sensed
And experienced by an audience
   As mental-emotional quiescence.

Light Verse on *Serious Themes*

1. Images of Equanimity

The act of rolling out
a painted Chinese scroll
inch by inch, gives action
to the stillness caught
by the artist's brush;
And adds the element of time
as scene by scene appears
in slow procession, visible instantly,
blending ending with
the entrance of a new beginning—
the composition of relationships
interacting tranquilly.

The Chinese art of exercise, T'ai-Chi Ch'uan,
creates a moving scroll of sculptured forms
unfolding subtly space by space
in empty air, only briefly visible.
And with the tempo's even pace,
the calligraphic style gives
ever changing sequences
a flowing continuity.
As each action-pattern creates a newer one,
it disappears, becoming choreographic memory

252   which, ingrained, keeps intact the essence
of the balanced harmony
of the structured forms.

Both painted scroll and moving scroll,
each in its own aesthetic way—
one with action in its stillness,
the other with stillness in its action—
Expressively evoke
the sentient spirit
of poise and equanimity.

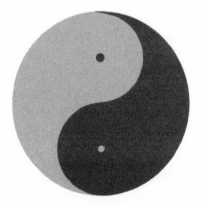

Ying Yang Balance

2. The Spirit of the Way in T'ai-Chi and the Ch'uan

The double-winged T'ai-Chi
give the Ch'uan's activity
an inexhaustible quantity
        of yin-yang certitudes.

Though tied to time and space
but never stratified, these certitudes
include a multitude
        of changing actions

which range from miniscule
fraction of the intangible,
        subtly present,
to the substantial
and totally felt tangible,
        deeply quiescent.

Without a starting point
or place of ending,
the T'ai-Chi's circling path—its boundary—
is limitless security
to wavelike energies within,

which flow from yin to yang
continuously in perpetuity.

> The core of its duality is—
> staying quiet with mobility
> seeming empty in activity
> appearing nonchalant with
> no concern, yet intent on
> every turn of place in space,
> feeling all maneuvers
> imperturbably.

The T'ai-Chi's inner
equanimity makes the outer
spirit of the Ch'uan
truly halcyon.

3. The Nine Elements:
A Trinity of Threes in the
Structure of T'ai-Chi Ch'uan

I. The "Organic Trinity"

Space-Time-Activity,
these organic threes,
an inseparable unity
indivisibly in motion,
function as a totality
with intrinsic amity.
> The universal way of timed-space
> and spaced-time activity, creates
> and bestows upon T'ai-Chi Ch'uan,
> the essential spirit
> of enduring harmony.

2. The "Personal" Trinity

These personal threes,
physical-mental-emotional,
as body, mind, and feeling
are individual entities
each aiding each without
losing its own identity.

The body is rudder-less
without mind's directions
yet it can keep the mind
from straying aimlessly;
with physical-mental interplay
emotions settle down unwittingly.
Life of the mind
is life with the body—
their harmony
is the home of equanimity.

3. The "Objective" Trinity

Form-Tempo-Movement,
these objective threes
interrelate proportionately
with the flow of yin-yang
energies interacting
at every living instant.
Form tempers tempo,
tempo shades movement,
movement shapes form,
These differing but never separated
elements, simultaneously active
in the "structure" of the personal threes—
give depth, meaning and
activity to the reality
of the "organic" trinity.

4. The Fourth Dimension

These nine elements
of the trinity of threes
coalesce spontaneously,
from which arises, unforeseen,

the tenth, far greater than the sum
of the integrated parts—
the element of containment—
      the state of feeling tranquil-calm
      while being vitally alert
      with the heightened awareness
      of the centered self—
a new dimension to experience.

4. A Three-Way Conversation

Mind Speaks Its Mind

If you, my body, ignore me, your mind,
I'll pay you back in kind.
I'll disappear, evaporate,
and leave you in a mindless state
of disarray, doomed to deteriorate
day by day as you meander
to and fro, hither and yon
moving like an automaton.
>Without a place for me
>in the heart of you,
>you'll act like a creature
>with a very low IQ.

But I have a true confession
to make—I, too, and many times I do,
forsake and abandon you—taking off,
unceremoniously, to far-off realms
of fantasy and subterranean thoughts,
leaving you to carry on, as best
you can, without the support
of a mentally guided plan.

I halt my selfish flight immediately
when, warned by your faltering activity
I sense the plight you're in—trying to function
without me, your mind's instruction.

I shall never stray away again
and neglect you, my body's presence.
Although I know that mind is
the essence of this exercise
I recognize objectively that
body-mind reciprocity
is the criterion for T'ai-Chi Ch'uan.

So when we both live on as constant friends
Then mutual confidence exists and conflict ends.

Emotion States Its Feelings

If you, my body, cooperate with mind
(and vice versa), I, your emotions,
will not nurse adverse feelings,
like anger, worry, fear, disquietude,
and any other mood of similar ilk.
I'll have instead, an even temperament,
as light and smooth as silk.

But should you, body, not be in accord
with mind (and vice versa), and go on
solo roads, it will bode ill for each of you.
I'll not be averse to lord it over you—
weakening body, upsetting mind—and, what's worse,
cause a commotion by expressing myself
with hyper-excessive emotion.

Body-mind, to you
I now appeal—let's make a deal.

If you will meet as one and try to be
constantly in complete rapport,
my good nature, from its deepest core,
will clearly be on its best behavior—
patient, calm, and steady,
ready to stay that way
(optimistically) forevermore.

The Body Expresses Itself

Where would you be, mind of mine,
without me, your body, to give you
a place to live and work in?
Probably lurking in some far-off space
trying to latch on to a wholesome soul
to match its body yang
with your own mental yin,
hoping for a new
dual cycle to begin.

Where in the world would I, your body, be
without you residing in me, guiding me?
Doubtless lulling listlessly, moving
in a groove of habitude, day by day
giving way to lassitude, without sense
or sensibility, in a state of debility.
What a destiny!

For the life of me
I cannot but see
that I thrive only
when you, my mind, are
alertly alive and "minding" me.
Unless you keep me close
as constant company, our feelings will

262   never be able to stay calm and stable
even on a very pleasant day.

Such awareness will inspire us
to aspire to levels higher
than the ordinary—for each of us
to become (it is a possibility) just
a wee bit more extraordinary.

5. Ch'i Explains Its Presence: Objectively

Let Ch'i tell you
what it is all about, since
it is an innate force that
no one in the whole wide world
can be alive without.

Though still a mystery, Ch'i
is a matter-of-fact
part of physiology
in partnership with breath
(without which—death).
The unity of yin and yang
(i.e., breath and Ch'i) makes
a longer span for living well
more than a possibility.

A life-giving force, Ch'i
is the source of energy
coursing through the system,
flowing and ebbing, in rhythm
with breathing and the body's form.

Normally a quiet presence
keeping breath close company,
Ch'i is stirred to rich activity
when the Mind decides to help it
do so (literally).

The Chinese way of exercise
to lead and feed the Ch'i
and reinforce its basic energy
is called Chi Kung.*
This technique sets the Mind,
(so to speak) "at the helm"
to regulate the tempo
and the depth of the breath
as well as to control all aspects
of the movements bodily.

The meeting of the conscious mind
with form and breath, instantly
raises the level
of Ch'i-energy.

In the exercise-art of T'ai-Chi Ch'uan,
where action moves on and on
continuously, mind is "one"
with form and respiration.
As in Ch'i-Kung methodology,
the combination of these three—
mind, breath, and physicality—
assures the increased flow
of life-force energy—the Ch'i—
insuring long-time health
and longevity.

Pronounced "tchee goong."

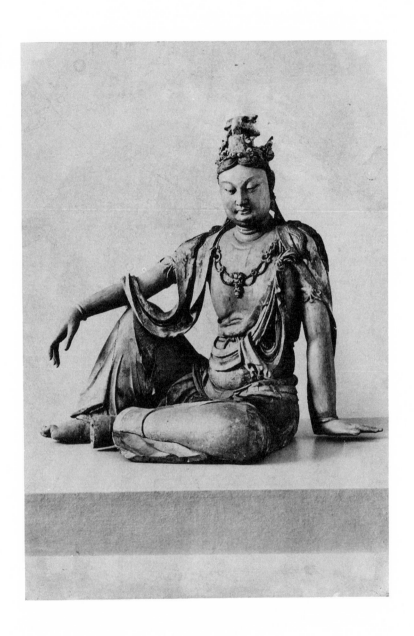

Containment

6. Aspects of Self-Awareness

At the Beginning—Becoming Still

At attention, light and easy,
     emptied of irrelevancies,
Full awareness of one's self.
Quietly alert, to sense
The moment before moving
     into space and form.

During Action—Moving Intrinsically

Differentiating subtleties
     link in constant flow;
Multi-units balance instantly,
Body-mind in unison,
Centering magnetically
     on every passing change.

At the Ending—Being Still

All is one, lightly soaring
     yet contained,
Filled with something
Other than before—
The presence of a tranquil present—
     serene, secure.

Feeling calm contentment
emptied of dilemmas,
Moving casually away
To normal functioning,
Clear-mindedly
with energies enriched.

7. The Way of T'ai-Chi Ch'uan

The body is alerted at every moment in a quiet way
> With the quiet way, energy is focused in
> balanced way

With the balanced way, heart-mind coordinates in a
perceptive way
> With perception, action is centered in a
> unified way

And with unity, mind-body functions in a tranquil way

In these light-hearted verses I am dealing with, in
popular fashion, principles which are present in the
philosophy and practice of T'ai-Chi Ch'uan.

1. "Thoughtless Thoughts"—Mind

2. "Instant Space"—Space and Time

3. "One over Two"—T'ai-Chi and Tao

4. The Nowness of the Now

Thoughtless Thoughts

When thoughts are really mean,
they bounce about like the
Mexican jumping bean,
        in their own dishevelled time,
        without rhyme or reason,
        as it pleases them.

When mind moves in to discipline
this disarray, they flutter off
to come again
        in quite another way, less
        maverick, as if to lull the mind
        to dull docility.

A minding mind cannot
be tricked so easily. Its will
can still the most distraught
        of thoughts—by being centered—
        thus freeing them, at best,
        from useless quests.

Instant Space

Cease grappling with curved concepts
      of time-space
      shaped by gravity.

Settle for illusions
that are with you
      realistically, not caring
      whether time is space or vice versa
      or that the place you take up
      makes a second, spacial.

Accept the status quo
of space and time rolled into one,
      until the time you can perceive spontaneously
      the spacelessness of time,
      the timelessness of space, or maybe
      non-space space or timeless time:

and until that time arrives
      to tell you each is neither—
      or the other—

Revel in this reality that
in the tiny space of a mini-moment
      you can unify
      space and time
      by the merest blink
      of your little eye.

One over Two

Taking a leaf from scholars
of various nations
and their differing interpretations
of the *Tao Te Ching* (Dow de Jing).
I venture now to bring
another view to you,
of T'ai-Chi (taiji) and the Tao (Dow).

The Tao is one, but as we know,
it is from two that all things grow
and multiply, even as you and I.

       Without the two of the T'ai-Chi
       where would the being of life be?

The Tao as one, removes the id
from identity making it nonentity
which then moves on to oblivion.

T'ai-Chi as two creates activity
resulting in a you and a me
for the sake of
a continuing humanity.

       But the world's duality
       was uni-formed by uni-verse
       and so informed that it was
       thus to be forevermore
          with Tao
          endowed.

The Nowness of the Now

The Now that is, is a Now that was
and Will-be as before it Was
and is to be—another past—

No sooner is Now is
than fast it goes to meet
a Will-be whose destiny will be
to be a Has-been immediately.

Without a mind to tell
the Now from Then and what makes
Will-be a reality, we'd dangle in the changeless Now-ness
of Infinity.

But since the changing chain of things that come and go,
remain forever in the stillness
of the brain, there is a possibility
that we can see, if only momentarily,
the Nowness of the Now—
anyhow.

8. The Essential Quality

The essential quality of T'ai-Chi Ch'uan
        is a way of moving
slowly, evenly, lightly,
continuously and in balance
        each form flowing into
the next with out stopping;
this creates a feeling
of calmness and ease.
        Patterns pass from one part
        of the body to the other
without strain and without
overworking a single part.
The heart never beats faster, nor
        is breathing quickened.
Attention centered on
the activity puts body
and mind into harmony.

9. A Message on Non-Violence to the Northeast Wind (The Yin and Yang of It)

It's true, dear northeast wind,
you blew the Peruvians
across the ocean
to Tahiti; but as for me,
          with your mighty
motion and your incessant
          din, you'll blow
          me into a loony bin.

               You penetrate my solid skin
               and spoil the quiet poise within.

Should I succumb to your wild activity
I'd become weak of body,
bleak of mind, and I'd wind up
          like the unkempt bush
and jittery tree, standing
at a forty-five degree angle
with my limbs and body
in an inextricable tangle.

Would I were a lofty palm
swaying gracefully, calm
in the face of your
misplaced force.

Your hoarse and fitful voices
never cease to go fortissimo
from screechy soprano to
basso profundo, raging,
bullying, bellowing
bellicosities like
Wall Street trading animosities.

Your strident sounds
and most erratic velocity
seem to boast that you
and only you can make
the world go round and round
and should you stop, the earth
would flop-drop, topple
into silent space
without a trace.

Dear trade wind, could you wander
less nomadically and visit us
sporadically, which you would do
if you knew that rushing around
madly from here to there will
get you nowhere in the
immeasurable atmosphere.

So calm down, windy, messy mass,
join the soul-saving intrinsic
class. When you cease moving
in the extrinsic way
you will save strength
for another day.

Dear noisy wind, with you as yang
and I as yin we'll never
begin to be a pair:
you are unseen air and
I am earthy real and can feel,
too often and too much,
your mighty touch.

Since we'll never be kin
while you are super yang
and I am ultra yin,
I shall always be contra you
unless I use my quietness
to conquer you.

I'll simply stuff my ears,
reduce you to a gentle hum.
With this strategy you will be a
lesser yang and I'll become a
fuller yin. Together then most
certainly we'll achieve
a modicum of equilibrium.

10. The Opposites Balance In the Chinese Theater

The cold vast theater is like a medieval fortress
Its stony walls cracked gray with time.
I sit encased in clothes uncomfortable
Immobile as a lump of clay
And fill the icy air with cloudy breath
While fast before me,
The actors fill the stage with warm activity
Swiftly as a summer storm, sommersault, and leap
And lightly as a gay balloon reach fingers to the skies
Then diving downward like a bird, feel earth
They toss and roll, as fluid as the flowing seas.

> Though frozen to my spot
> I free my body from its weighted folds
> And bare my fingers to the freezing air
> Made hot by such lightheartedness.

The vast hot theater is like a medieval dungeon,
Its walls of stone drip wet with tropic heat.
I sit as thinly clad as custom will allow
And fan the air with passive energy
As listless as a fly at summer's end

While easily before me they jump and dash around
As turbulent as interrupted bees
And cooly, with the calm of Kuan Yin seated in a shady cave,
They whirl their massive robes and twirl their spears.

Though hotly rooted to my spot
I drink the boiling tea with love
And lightly toss my futile fan away
Made cool by such intensity

L'Envoi

A dancer's art brings ease in wintertime,
A dancer's art brings ease in summertime.

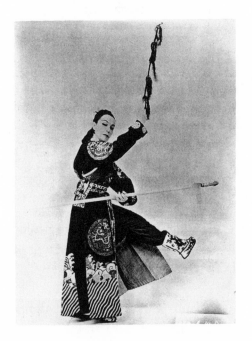

**Fig. 9.1 The Classical Chinese Theater.
(Copyright © Sophia Delza.)**

11. A Friendly Way

T'ai-Chi Ch'uan, a Chinese exercise-art
Has had a very early historic start
      and continues—for any nationality—
      to be a path to longevity
With mindfulness a long-lasting part.

The exercise-art of T'ai-Chi Ch'uan
will give life's span a long, long run
      with mind and body harmony.
      This almost is a certainty
when T'ai-Chi Ch'uan practice is properly done.

T'ai-Chi Ch'uan is the friendly way
To travel with each and every day
      Acquiring strength and fortitude
      and an easy stable mood
which comes from balanced yin-yang interplay.

CHAPTER X

THE EXPANDING SCOPE OF AWARENESS

Infinite in its effect is change
Of matter due to T'ai-Chi action.
No trace of tension shows in energy
Dynamic balance conquers strain and stress.
Vitality is free from nervousness
And strength evolves with pliancy
Attention centered on the action
Kindles patience, poise, tranquility
And equilibrium in continuum.

Satisfaction with oneself
is not enough; the centered being
Sensitized, includes a circle
Larger than the self; the silent sounds
Of T'ai-Chi Ch'uan reverberate
With essence of responsibility
To conduct, work, and daily life,
To do as well as think and be
is an intrinsic necessity.

The Expanding Scope of Awareness

1. The Art of the Science of T'ai-Chi Ch'uan

In the science of T'ai-Chi Ch'uan lies the definite knowledge of how man can best regulate himself in all aspects of living—physically, emotionally, mentally. In the art of T'ai-Chi Ch'uan lies the process that produces a state of harmonious well-being and, with this, the realization that man can achieve and experience a unique sense of emotional and mental integration.

The science and the art are inseparable and are experienced simultaneously. Both function through a technique which is dominated by a *way*, a textured way of moving that determines the effect of this multifaceted composition. This way is embedded in the very nature of its aims (its science), and it is the cause of the essential inner experience and the outer expression (its art).

This exercise-art, the antithesis of the accidental, the unpremeditated, the blindly inspirational, is composed, ordered, figured out, developed according to theory, thought, philosophy, science, mathematics, and the laws of nature.

T'ai-Chi Ch'uan is an ancient Chinese system of exercise which activates the body for the superior development of physical, emotional, and mental well-being. Constructed according to the physiological laws of body-behavior, it is motivated by a philosophy based on the assumption that the complete personality can be involved in, and therefore can benefit in a multitude of ways from a physical activity directed by the mind with awareness.

An ancient exercise, it goes back to the late twelfth century when it is said to have been completed, indicating, of course, that its roots reach far back in China's history. In one of the earliest books on health, the *Nei Ching* (Canon of Medicine, c. 300 B.C.E.), the search for a harmonious way of life included not only medical and hygienic techniques but also ethical and philosophic values.

T'ai-Chi Ch'uan is the accumulation and culmination of a thousand years of thought and experimentation on how the body can best develop its intrinsic and potential qualities. Widely practiced in China today, it has remained substantially the same in motivation, although its forms have changed over the centuries, as any art must, in order to stay related to growing cultures, and creative and scientific developments.

The structure of T'ai-Chi Ch'uan is symphonic in length, being at its minimum twenty-two minutes long, to be continuously executed with no stopping at any point. Comprised of 108 Forms and composed to the last detail in space and time, the exercise is a uniquely structured whole—a moving three-dimensional mural. Each Form is a subtle climax of multiple designs and movements with varying dynamics and relationships. The entire organization is so harmoniously balanced in terms of its parts and its purposes that it can not but be included in the sphere of art, including as it does concern with space, shape, and object as in painting, and motif, space, time as in music and dance.

The concrete material of this physical exercise correlates all of man's faculties as he puts his body into action, his mind into awareness, and his spirit into serenity. Compose the body and the mind is calmed; settle the mind and the emotions are composed. The thought, the feeling, the action—each can be the root, the link, the cause, and the effect. Whichever the way, the result is a balance of the vital energy of body and mind.

Although this composition is not an original for anyone, the participator, in reenacting the structure, creates it anew, so to speak, and is transformed by it. He himself becomes the work of art in the doing of it. Comprehension of what he is doing, and the awareness of what it is, makes it possible for him to achieve the harmony of physical security, emotional ease, mental poise, and, what is essential to the spirit of T'ai-Chi Ch'uan, to experience its aesthetic quality.

It is the science of its structure based on the natural laws of body-behavior and action that produces the power of sustained good health. It is the art that creates the heart-mind (in Chinese—*hsin*) ease, its containment (emotional), and contentment (aesthetic).

The emotional-aesthetic feeling is not at all like the peaceful pleasure that comes from listening to great music, or from seeing a great painting. It is not the same as the satisfaction or joy that a creative artist (in any medium) derives while working, or experiences at the conclusion of his *chef-d'oeuvre*—although this latter feeling, if it comes from his *art* and not from his finishing it, might faintly approach, in heart-mind ease, the special feelings aroused by T'ai-Chi Ch'uan. The dancer experiences another kind of joy from her performance of her own created dances—a dynamic aliveness caused by emotional physical stimula. For all of these arts, it is the observer, the audience, as recipient of the finally finished art, who experiences the aesthetic reaction.

With T'ai-Chi Ch'uan it is the doer, the performer of this masterpiece, who reacts to the art of this art at the same time as he becomes the art; he *is* as he lives it in space and from moment to moment. The onlooker, the observer is not needed for the aesthetic completion of this work of art. He may become engrossed by it and may detect its artistic nature, and although he may (possibly) understand it, he cannot *feel* its intrinsic nature which is part of its art; but because he cannot benefit from the *function* of its form, he cannot have the true aesthetic experience.

When I first saw T'ai-Chi Ch'uan being practiced in the T'ai Miao Park in Peking (1948), I already knew something about the dynamically expressive style and content of the Classical Chinese Theater; I had seen many examples of the Chinese folk-character dancers, which were gay, blithe, charming. Being a dancer, I am well acquainted with many dance styles as well as with various exercise-techniques. But the impact of T'ai-Chi Ch'uan on me was one of such unusual power that I knew it could not be measured by any already learned standards, however profound.

The beauty of the flow of movement seemingly effortless, the harmonious designs of the interlacing forms, and the calm composition as balanced as the horizon made me feel, on first seeing, that my aesthetic perceptions were not those of an outsider. With longer looking, however, there gradually crept into my consciousness faint apprehension of my ignorance, that there was more to it than met my eye, and that my knowledge was quite limited. After a time of watching, I could surmise that the doer was experiencing from the process of action something—a sense of being—which could not be projected outward to affect the observer similarly; that what I was experiencing was an awareness of its art-nature and not the aesthetic nature of its art, which came from the doing and not from the seeing, as I was to discover from personal experience.

The nature of its art is what I am analyzing in this essay: what I eventually came to learn, from doing and comprehending it, to be the essence of this balanced exercise system, and why T'ai-Chi Ch'uan is as fine an art as are any of our customary fine arts, even though it is a complete art for the doer alone and only a secondary art for the observer.

Inevitably we have an art when the harmonious blending of form and function arouses a special feeling in the observer as in the fine arts, and, as I believe, when it produces a state of being in the doer, as in T'ai-Chi Ch'uan.

A distinction has been made, in Chinese history, between the art of exercise (personal-philosophic) and the art of dance (philosophic-communal). To stir and stimulate the mind and emotions of the observer through designed body-action was the province of dance-art, whether it was, as in very ancient times, ritualistic or commemorative; whether it was dramatic personification as done in what I call early theater, or folk, court, and theater dance in more recent centuries. Those designed body movements created to stir and stimulate the mind, the emotions, and the *body* of the doer himself have been called health, medical, or hygiene gymnastics or exercise. This may appear to us an obvious distinction, but exercise in Western terms is rarely if ever thought of as being an art in the symbolic sense of the word, not in the literal sense—that of doing. All the Chinese exercises I know (several classes and styles) I consider art because they incorporate the aesthetic dimentions of fine art in their compositions.

In judging any art certain fundamentals must inevitably be considered. When we speak of music, dance, theater, painting, or sculpture, we include in our analysis and critical judgments the totality of the composition, the significance of the form, the quality of technical execution, rhythmic consistency, vitality of idea and pattern, dynamics of movement and space, and the special values inherent in the separate arts: color in painting, tone and time in music, and space-time-movement in dance, and a complex of values in the theatrical art—speech, movement, design, direction.

Art, without purpose or direction, without motivation for the form, generally results in being mechanically formal (abstract expressionism included). Subject matter, no matter how important, will never alone make an art art-worthy; it must be significantly expressed in terms of the art medium. In T'ai-Chi Ch'uan, form and function are so totally integrated that function acts through the form, and form reveals and becomes the function. Complete synthesis produces what I call a fourth dimension, the aesthetic content.

How do we get an art aesthetic from such fusion? For me, art is greater than the sum of its parts, function and method, function and form. The expression of a concept-emotion-idea which inspires the artist is rendered by form, comprising arrangement, structure, pattern, design, rhythm, dynamics, all of which is the third dimension, so to speak. The greater dimension that *is* the art-aesthetic is the by-product of the fusion of form and concept. If this art product is successful, this fourth dimension comes into being: it is this that is its artistic aesthetic nature, its art content. I say, therefore, that it is greater than the sum of its parts because something new has come into existence, born of thought and technique. The subject-motive determines form-motif and the union creates a special art-content. The science of the form-function of T'ai-Chi Ch'uan has produced an art for the one who enacts it; for the observer, it sympathetically produces a state of awareness of the existence of an art and arouses in him, empathetically, a state of repose.

I find it convenient for art analysis to use the ABCs to denote Architecture-arrangement, Body-behavior (techniques), and Concept-content. In T'ai-Chi Ch'uan the ABCs occur all in one; their union takes place at every moment, so that when discussing one aspect I am inferring a direct connection and inner relationship with the others.

The way of the movement, the body technique, and the space design and body configurations are absolutely the consequence of the goals and benefits to be derived from performing the complete exercise daily. There is no vagueness about the principles for self-development. To improve the body's health, physical skill, and stamina is to increase the possibility for longer life. The ability to concentrate and coordinate and to deepen mental perceptivity and alertness produces quicker reflexes, awareness, observation, and control, and therefore greater harmony of thought and action. Coordination of mind and body is conducive to calmness, without which no one can be considered truly healthy. Such harmony (with which to function more astutely in no matter what field of work) and the exploring of qualities deep in man not yet awakened, these are the concepts which had inspired various Chinese philosophers to devote their lives to the creation of an exercise art which would realize these goals. Chang San Feng of the late Sung dynasty, twelfth century, is said to be the final creator of T'ai-Chi Ch'uan, having spent most of his ninety years in the philosophically scientific, according to nature's plan, exploration of these ideas.

Since T'ai-Chi Ch'uan is a discipline of body movement, it can be shown by concrete analysis how the form functions and how the function forms the action. It must be remembered that whatever is said of any action, though treated separately, each relates at all times to the three centers of mind, body, and emotion.

Regardless of whether patterns are intricate or simple, whether motions are parallel or opposite, whether positions are high or low, diagonal or straight, the following fundamental qualities are irrevocably present: (1) the tempo is slow in accordance with a good heartbeat, with natural breathing, and neither is ever speeded up; (2) movement is continuous and flowing with no interruption; (3) except for nine momentary places, movement is never overcome by the force of longevity, meaning that the body is always in physical balance; (4) the dynamics of light and strong (yin and yang) are always in a state of continual change, moving as gradually as day shades into night and night into day, including the fulfilled climaxes of each.

Substance of this movement-art is in the Form: how it comes into being; how it is completed; how it changes and becomes another Form.

Substance is in the Action: it is the working relationship between muscles and joints; it is the transformation of a transition to a Form; it is the texture (yin-yang) of the movement. This substance is "controlled yet airy in appearance"; it has "the stillness of a mountain and the agility of a river"; it contains the spirit of the concentrated alertness of "a cat waiting to catch a mouse"; and it has the form in potential speed of "a hawk trying to snatch a rabbit." The collective aspect of substance contributes to the fine art of this exercise-art.

Form forms the space; time shapes the patterns; and space times the Forms. The ingredients of shape, space, time (tempo), pattern, direction, and substance are factors continually at play in such impeccable relationships that (1) the body, internally and externally, is in perfect equilibrium; (2) the yin-yang elements are proportionately related; (3) unity in every active moment is apparent despite the complexity of changes. It is a world of changing unities.

Each of the 108 Forms is a culmination of a variety of designed movements with ever-changing dynamic tones. Each is felt as an inevitable tangible resolution of a chain of interweaving intangible transitions. A Form is a synchronized frame or chord of completion in a not-visible halt.

To overcome the inertia caused by the static nature of the Form, the mind must be especially alert to send the body into action. The mind must be present at every moment in T'ai-Chi Ch'uan, which is called a "from the mind" exercise. Conscious concentration directs the movements as a result of which interfering irrelevant thoughts are eliminated. But, especially, it is when action becomes familiar and habitual that the mind has a tendency to blank itself out or wander away. It is this that the organization of the designs of T'ai-Chi Ch'uan prevents.

It is so easy for the body to become an automaton and act out of blind habit, to its own detriment. For instance, in acting, the mind must be present to help the actor to relive his often repeated words and movements, thus each time imbuing the most familiar sequences with fresh life, otherwise the action and lines would take over and the result would be mechanical, without heart or intelligence.

The discipline of making the mind stay with one is an intrinsic part of the structure of this exercise. It can never be walked through; it must be lived through each time. This develops a mental alertness that becomes part of everyday living and working. With true awareness which gives security, self-consciousness or emotional ill-ease will *never* intrude on the consciousness.

The following is an illustration of the way the structure forces mental activity and informs one of being in a mental blank-out. Whenever a Form is repeated, it proceeds to a new design, a new arrangement. Should the mind be elsewhere, wandering around away from the subject at hand, an early habit will take over and make the body move into a previously made position; it is interesting to note that as soon as this happens, in this technical structure, something stirs in the mind and the mistake is recognized. The structure of repeated sequences is so arranged that they never take place in the same floor space. This fact is also a means to call attention to a variation and to a mistake. Actually every momentary change is a problem for the mind. The interrelation of mind directing the changes and of the changes waking up and prodding the mind is ever present.

What happens in space is never accidental nor arbitrary, mainly because man's physiological structure determines the design, that is, every movement affects the shape of the space. Accurately made space directions will help to improve the body's form by way of joint articulations. Correctly made body positions will take place in the designated areas. Structure can be manipulated by space placement; space can adjust the forms. If a stance is incorrect, because of the improper body position, for example, hips thrust out in back forcing the leg and spine alignment to be wrong, the change of movement in space will not work. If the spatial design is wrong, for example, too widely or narrowly spaced, the body will not be able to move correctly into the next specific design. The body checks the space and the space the body's unity. To understand this is to see the total unification of inner and outer structures, the interfusion of science of the body and the art of its use in space, the juxtaposition of the tangible and intangible, and the harmony of self in action in relation to static environment.

The observer responds agreeably to the manifest inevitability of movement sequences—a coming out in the right place at the right time; this is harmony of space and form. The observer does not have to wait for a resolution of a series of movements and a climax of ideas, because the idea exists at every moving movement, visibly. For the doer, the accumulation of these moments over a 22–25 minute period is another matter and of greatest significance, since the most valuable effect of T'ai-Chi Ch'uan lies in its length, just as eating the whole apple is more salutory for the body's needs than a single bite, as the greater benefits are contained in and attained from the accumulation of the Forms, although each unit is composed of the ingredients of the whole.

The floor pattern the feet traverse is as exact as a mathematical equation. The enclosing shape is that of a rectangle, the side to side (east and west) width being fourteen foot-lengths long, each individual's foot size, not the standard 12-inch measurement, determining the distance. The front to back (north and south) length is seven foot-lengths long. The east-west axis line comes between the second and third foot-lengths. The starting *and* the finishing space is at the same point, being at the fourth step in from the right (east) with the toes touching the axis line. It must be said here that the off-center placement is typical for all symmetrical postures, of which there are not many. A symmetrical position is fairly static and coming as it does away from a centered point, its immobile effect is diminished, while its restful effects are augmented (Fig. 10.1.)

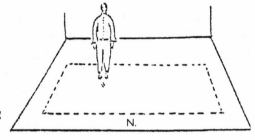

Fig. 10.1 The Starting Point

The floor space "walkings" go in eight directions which are called, like the points of the compass, north, east, south, west, and northeast, northwest, southeast, southwest (for philosophic as well as practical reasons). The awareness of space is three-dimensional, however, with a height of seven foot-lengths for the exercise volume, forming a space like a double cube. The four upper and four lower diagonal corners, as angled from the torso itself, are important in respect to body design and space structure. Every person recognizes the limits of his own 7 by 14 by 7 (in height) volume, even when the exercise is done outdoors.

It can be seen that such complexity of direction is more than moving the feet along a path, but this directional aspect is absolutely simple compared to the multitude of changes the body is capable of even in that confined space. And these changes and variations, though complex, are *not* uncalculated—they have been chosen, regulated, selected, devised by *plan* which adheres to the intent (as function) and to the essential principles (as form).

Combined meaningfully as they are (in every unit of action) with every angle of the 360 degree circle, and with every structural requirement of body in space scrupulously considered, it can be appreciated how scientifically profound and artfully astute were the philosophic creators of T'ai-Chi Ch'uan—the more so because nothing is abstracted from meaning, although the method is objective and universal.

Before getting into the practical and tangible explanation of how the Forms and their "formings" are balanced—by means of line, space, shape, dynamics, depth, volume—it must be stated here that the textured way of movement, as I called it earlier, is by far the most important technique to carry out specific goals. Aesthetically, this moving way is easily the most apparent of all the techniques and has the greatest effect on the onlooker; and it is the most difficult to achieve. This way is the continuity in movement which builds up endurance; it is the subtlety of moving the joints (to link up form) which develops keen perceptivity; it is the never-stopping, endless flow which increases control; it is itself calm, evoking calmness—which improves concentration.

The way of smoothly sustained movement is described (in the T'ai-Chi Ch'uan Canon, fifteenth century) as resembling "the even control (in pulling) required to draw out the silk thread from a cocoon"; to pull jerkily would break the thread; to pull too lightly is ineffectual. To achieve the correct technique, the mind must be centered and control the activity. The accomplishment of mind-body unity creates a sense of tranquillity which, inwardly felt, is radiated outward.

The way of holding the muscles comes from the structure itself, just as carrying a heavy or light load demands a different degree of energy expended. In T'ai-Chi Ch'uan all changes of intensities are never made visibly, never externalized. This is an intrinsic exercise: changes of force result from the designs and forms themselves, so that muscular variations are built-in, therefore invisible (but, of course, greatly felt). The muscular effort needed to stand on one leg is as little seen as is the lesser stress used to stand on two legs; a deep knee pose seems to take no more energy than the lifting of a light arm. What makes this concealed effort possible is the way the movements move into each other through joint action, by the balance of the structural sequences as they relate to space, and by the fact that the alternation of yin and yang dynamics is microscopically graduated, giving the body time to adjust itself intrinsically to the changing forms.

The way of the formation of the Forms and transitions is circular—the "going" is curvilinear, as are the spiral, loop, oval, crescent, parabola, and, a circle or any part thereof. There are, according to my way of thinking, two classes of curve: the natural physical way, and the designed, created, curvilinear motion.

The body cannot but move in curves of varying degrees; this is the natural way. Here we see, more obviously than elsewhere, the principle of working with and from nature first, and then evolving elaborations from it, in a sense becoming supernatural. Lift an arm from a low point to a higher one and an arc is described, making a segment of a circle. Pivoting on the heel, toes move, and an arc is made, much in the same way as does a compass. When the body turns in space it makes a circling. This is a natural law of body in space.

The designed curve is a creative extension of this physiological fact, and a necessary addition since the main purpose of
this exercise is to augment the natural condition of body and
mind far beyond the capacities we were born with. Because of
our very complexity, the nature of the circular action must cor-
respondingly be extended far above the natural, yet, as can be
seen, always working with, in tune with, the natural.

From the fact that the beginning Form and the ending
Form are at the same place, we can perceive the architectural
space to be in the form of a circle, with the diagonal directions
to be considered as segments, a circle within a rectangle. Our
rectangular (so to speak) body describes spatial circles at every
turn, low or high, right or left, rectangle within a circle.

Structurally speaking, the curve is everywhere: in the
natural turn of a wrist and in the designed half-circle of an arm
gesture; in the natural turn of a head and in the designed wavelike motion of retreating or advancing movement. A complex
combination of a parabolic curve of an arm, timed with a half-
turn of a wrist, as the head turns and dips, with the leg making
a hooklike pattern, this is typical of the variety of design and
curve that appears throughout the exercise. And not to lose
sight of its function—such action develops coordination and
stability, awareness and perception of the subtle (Fig. 10.2.)

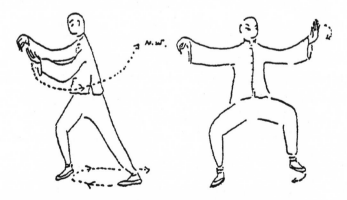

Fig. 10.2 The Curving Movements of the Transitions

The curve shades motion and stillness from the most obvious actions to the most delicate refinements—like the movements of a wave propelling itself into, and therefore making, another wave. Ability to balance at every conceivable moment is made possible by the curved-way action. The circular way prevents expenditure of energy and reserves strength to be used only when needed. In the process of doing the exercise, the expended moment of finality, like "the shooting or letting-go of the arrow," is never part of the action. Rather, the body feeling is like that of the drawing of the bowstring, always ready to take off, alive, poised, concentrated and aware and reserved, ready for the final release. The curved way with its wavelike, to-and-fro, give-and-take dynamics contributes to the resilient activity of muscles, which method gives the body elasticity and pliability.

A circle embraces one with security, and distils containment. The concept of the circle creates stillness and calmness. And contained as the multiple complexities are within it, the result is a balance of the two forces of activity and stillness.

The T'ai-Chi shape symbolizes the containment of the continuous flow of energy which, according to universal principles, is of two kinds, the yin and the yang. These two opposite forces, to cite some examples, like ebb and flow, diastole-systole, negative-positive, stillness-movement, female-male, backward-forward, moon-sun, earth-heaven, and so on, balance and partner each other, never in opposition, but always as complements; the indisputable fact is that we cannot and do not have one without the other. In this T'ai-Chi symbol, the inference is that each, containing as it does a touch of the other (yin in yang, yang in yin), dissolves into and evolves from the other with complete and irrefutable consistency, based as it is on the fact that there is nothing without change in the universe (Fig. 10.3.)

This point of view explains and is reflected both in the palette, the muscle-tone coloration in movement-technique, and in the changing formations of the structure. The palette is limited by the natural organic process of energy changes required by the structural forms. This is the T'ai-Chi way. The lightest tone

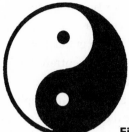

Fig. 10.3 The T'ai-Chi Symbol

is light to that degree of tension which keeps the body in control and active. In the entire exercise there is never any relaxed (succumbing to gravity) position, as, for instance, a loose head or a limp hand on an outstretched arm would be. Every movement is contemplated, directed, and controlled. The strongest muscular tension results from intrinsic form and not from subjective extraneous manipulation, such as *tensing* the fist to exhibit strength. The body is always capable of *more* strength than it shows or ever uses. But the extent of the dynamics is nevertheless very great indeed, as the movement moves from the lightest tone of a simple gesture to very complicated positions demanding great inner force to make and hold them. Because of such intrinsic restraints, and because the circular way dominates the shape-form, the external appearance of all the action seems effortless and weightless.

These sensations of lightness and strength are felt internally. Seen are the moving relationships of ever-changing structure; never seen is the passage of power that causes them. Here is a simple description of the contrast of what is felt and what is seen, and can be easily experienced by the reader. Raise your arms forward up to shoulder level; arms are parallel with straight wrists; palms face downward. Here the muscles of the arms and hands feel light. Without moving the arms out of this position move your hands so that the fingers point to the ceiling and the palms face forward: the action of putting and keeping the hands in this position activates the arm muscles very forcefully. Then lower the hands to the original position and feel the release of muscle pressure. What can be seen is a change of form; what is felt is a change of power, as well as the gradual dynamic change. If you move the hands slowly and concentrate to perceive the muscles' gradual differences, you will appreciate in an elementary way the possibility of dynamic textures in complicated action.

Never undertensed beyond control, never tensed beyond equilibrium (for the form), the doer can achieve, by these means, the ends of endurance and awareness, sensitive perception, and stable energy.

Creating a work of art is more than a mathematical process. For instance, to arrive at the number ten, one must have the proper digits, but they can be arranged in no-matter-what order. For a work of art, not only must all the components be there but, what is most important, their order and arrangement must be profoundly considered to achieve the art—the artistic and the desired effect. In T'ai-Chi Ch'uan the Forms, progressing and evolving through a complex path of structure, tempo, and dynamics accomplish their goals by the collective force of selected ingredients (science) and their compositional arrangement (art), finally arrived at by those Chinese philosophers who had knowledge of the life of nature and the nature of life.

The human being has an irrevocable Form, the subtleties of which vary in each individual. Though T'ai-Chi Ch'uan is an arranged structure, it is no stereotype. Just as the personal foot-length regulates the traversed distance of the floor area, so does the individual's body proportions determine the balance of the configurations made with torso, arms, and legs around itself. But the patterned movements themselves are mathematically directed in external terms, as in the angled degree in which the figure turns in any of the eight directions, in the placement of the foot in 45, 90, or 135 degree angles, and so on. The composition itself is exactly determined and designed, as to where the arms, legs, knees, and head are to be moved; but the individual's physique will subtly determine the degree of the body curve and knee-bend action, or the height of a raised leg.

However, the balanced result in each and every person must be the same: the same, let us say, as a circle is a circle whether it is small or large. In the Forms and their formings, the process is quite complicated since each moment of moving involves tempo, space, structure, yin-yang dynamics, balance, stillness, and activity, which make the totality.

Figure 10.2 illustrates the various points in the above paragraph. In the Single Whip Form, the heels are separated from each other by the length of two paces, a space that differs for people with different foot sizes. The depth to which the knees bend depends on personal ability and flexibility, too; but the body attitude is the same for all—the knees must be in line with the toes, the torso and waist must be in correct position, the toes must point to the stipulated compass angles, and the entire direction of the Form must be exact in terms of external space. This is an example of the personal self being disciplined objectively. Because of the logic of our common organic structure, such objective discipline does not violate our personalities. And because of our individualistic natures there is never to be seen any chorus-like uniformity. Rather, through the regulated order and perfection of the moving postures, the individual's capacities, sensibilities, and abilities are heightened and sensitized.

The elements of structure in any single pattern are balanced, balanced in terms of gravity, dynamics, space, and form; all are resolved proportionately in minute measurements and in exact ratio, so that at every moment peaceful harmony is felt and conveyed.

What happens in the distribution of size and weight, strength and lightness is obviously clear when we take as an example a pound of feathers, which takes a large space, and balance it with a pound of iron, which takes up a small space. In T'ai-Chi Ch'uan when a leg design is light (hsu—void), the space covered is greater than its balancing counterpart which is compact (shih—solid), and the rest of the body will be patterned with varying degrees of lightness and strength, making complete unity.

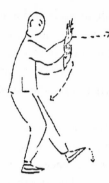

Fig. 10.4 The Hand Strums the Lute Form

In Hand Strums the Lute (Fig. 10.4), the right leg with bent knee is solid, carrying most of the weight, and the left leg, outstretched, rests lightly on the heel, covering as much ground as the length of leg permits. The right arm with palm turned outward (yang) is strongly centered halfway toward the chest, and the left arm with palm inward (yin) is lightly placed outside of right so that fingers reach right wrist. The larger space of light left arm balances the smaller space of the stronger right arm, as do the legs: the light left covers a large space and the strong right is in small body space.

So impeccably balanced is each moving Form that "a single feather added to one's body and a false movement would destroy the balance." Placing the left hand, for instance (in Fig. 10.4.), inside the right-hand space would feel as awkward as hearing a wrong note struck in a familiar phrase. The measure of the changing weight balances the power and makes the power of balance: power is not force; it is the ability to control.

Every Form and process can be analyzed, each with its own sum of balances. The flow of movement is also securely balanced at each fractional second. As has been mentioned, the dynamics cannot be seen because of their intrinsic nature. In the interweaving and dovetailing of pattern into pattern, the proportion of space to space is never *not* right. Arrangement and dynamics, space-size and the textured way, are correlated much in the same way as a colorist would harmonize the pale or brilliant, the dark or light hue in respect to space and juxtaposition in organizing his canvas to express his ideas.

In T'ai-Chi Ch'uan, however, since it is a moving canvas, the transitions, transmitted like the perpetual flow of a river, displace and alter each situation so skillfully that depth and space, framework and Form, appear and disappear with singular ease. With such a method, the mind is always intrigued, the power of the action stabilized, and the element of calmness increased.

The greater the balance, the lighter is the look. The more fluid the transitions, the less visible is the technique which in turn is then more proficient. Seen is the design, the action, the activity of structural and directional changes in relation to each other and to a "still part," that part of the body which does not change its position. Without a point of reference, a point of contrast, so much activity as has been described could become excessive and produce restlessness, in terms of T'ai-Chi Ch'uan principles (not necessarily in terms of art-dance).

In the course of changing (with a few exceptions), some part of the body is momentarily still. I analyze *stillness* as being of three kinds: (1) as related both to body and to space; (2) as related to space; (3) as related to body. The first is most easily seen and done. A stance is taken and legs and torso remain still while the arms, head, fingers move. This is activity taking place

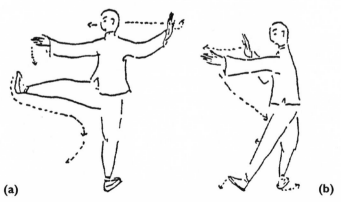

(a)　　　　　　　　　　　　　　　　　　(b)

Fig. 10.5 Stillness vis-à-vis the Body and Space

in an obviously held position. Here we have control and rest at the same time (Fig. 10.5a.)

Second, stillness in relation to space means that one part of the body is kept in the same geometric relationship to space despite movement in the rest of the body. In the Form where the left leg is sidewards and the left arm is parallel to the floor, the left arm will remain in this parallel-space position all the time, while the left and right knees bend, thus lowering the torso and while the torso turns to face east (Fig. 10.5b.)

Third, stillness in relation to the body means that a particular part does not move from its position in relation to the body, while its geometric place in space is being changed by movement in *another* part of the body. In The Stork Flaps Its Wings, the right arm, circled around the head, remains fixed in this position while the torso bends, twists, and rises (Fig. 10.6.)

The still or suspended movement forms an aspect of space design that demands a new control. The ability to isolate and control any part of the body in its context with the planned Form is another unique way to elevate the standard of coordination in both body and mind. From a purely physical standpoint, such nonaction gives more power to resist the pull of gravity. We already saw examples of sets of muscles exercised not by themselves moving but by action in a connected part. (A simple illustration would be that of moving the torso and shoulders

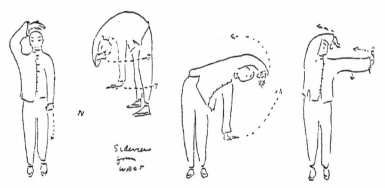

Fig. 10.6 The Stork Flaps His Wings Form

around to each side while keeping the head still, to exercise the neck muscles.)

Visually and physically, the design of action contrasted with a still motif becomes more and more complex, especially when gestures move in opposition. Add to this the fact of subtle tempo variations, and the possibility for multiple subrelationships of themes increases enormously.

Space form determines tempo, and the tempo shapes the space. The original and basic tempo, decided upon by the opening gesture, is always present, being carried by some part of the moving body at all times. This basic tempo controls the form and dominates the movement in space. But within this basic tempo are slower tempos of varying lesser speeds.

To illustrate tempo and form synchronization, I use the familiar example of the minute and second hands of a clock, both of which arrive at their destined moment together, making a unity of sixty seconds and one minute. This action is smooth, regular, precise. In the execution of certain Forms, a similar but more complicated synthesis takes place, because some part of the body may be moving at a different tempo.

Since each Form is a synchronized moment, it is inferred that all parts of the body have to arrive at their appointed places at the same moment. Some parts will have had to move over large or small areas, therefore taking different time periods to culminate the Form simultaneously. The rule is that the basic tempo is maintained by the part moving in the largest space. The tempo used in the smaller spaces is always slowed down, the degree of slowness depending on the relative distances, as, for example, an arm moving in a quarter circle will have to slow down by half the tempo taken by an arm making a half circle, if they are to meet at the same place, together.

From a position where the body and legs are still, the crossed hands must move to meet at the left ear; the right arm makes a large circle at the same time that the left makes a short arc to reach the place. The right arm maintains the basic tempo, while the left moves more than twice as slowly. This is a broad example of tempo differences. When areas have less differentia‑ tion, the degrees of tempo changes are delicate indeed. The orchestration of arms, legs, torso, head, turning, lowering and lifting, going forward and backward, demands a deep perception of time as well as structure. The proportions of the flowing pic‑ tures must be controlled with concentration and patience. The feeling of calm comes from accuracy, and mental enrichment comes from the varying complexities. The greater the perfection of synchronization the more the enjoyment, the more profound the perception, the richer the experience of the art.

The wonder of T'ai-Chi Ch'uan is the lack of clock-time feeling despite such specific delineations of time and space. The objective feeling of a vacuum of time arises from the unending continuity of the moving process, from the "seamlessness" of the interlacing forms, and especially from the constancy of balance— the composite order of all which produces a state of weightless‑ ness in the body (and of no-limit to the psyche).

Comprehension of the composition as a whole is appre‑ ciated only after all the individual units, which are small totali‑ ties, have been learned in unaltered sequence. It is the reverse of how we generally come to understand a picture, where first we look for the dominating structure or the central theme, after which we analyze the detailed elements. In T'ai-Chi Ch'uan, because each idea-unit is complete in itself and leads with con‑ sistency into another unit, perception grows with the experience of relating them to each other. It is when the small total Forms are comprehended that the larger masses which embrace them can be recognized as being made up of the same forces, but fashioned less obviously and more ingeniously. Consciousness of the greater structures increases the aesthetic appreciation of the scientific whole.

The exercise is divided into six series, each of which is quite individual as to character, and different (here described only in broad outline) as to: spatial planning and the main lines of direction-advancing in series 1, and retreating in series 2; the demands made on energy for balancing in series 3; the levels of coordination and concentration in series 4; the psychological devices of the use of repeated themes in series 5; introduction of new themes until the very last moment of action to keep attention and interest from flagging in series 6. Each section has its unique group of Forms, stimulating the mind and using the body in special ways.

What is seen and felt in the microcosm is appreciated and experienced in the macrocosm, but on a large scale and in different proportions: alternation of opposite forces like bending-straightening, forward-backward, opening-closing, in-out, up-down, powerful-easy, complex-simple, and so forth; changing weight dynamics; variety in Form and Tempo; ebb and flow in movement sensation; variations in design so that the body never tires. The facts of balance and of continuous movement are innate, as is the never-ending, never-ceasing flow, so that the division between any two series is never visible.

Even with such a variegated process of multiple patterns within Forms, and Forms within series, there is never a touch of superfluity in pattern, design, movement; no unneeded gesture, no decoration ever appears. Even in the most strenuous of positions, no superfluous demands are made upon the body. With the technique of learning to "lift a pound with a pound of energy," all movements are true to use, consistent, never awkward, therefore beautiful.

The most minute turn of every gesture is selected, every action is chosen and combined according to the intrinsic laws of how the body functions best, and to the limitations set by the age-old objectives based on mental and physical balance and emotional equanimity. It is inevitable that artistry should grow out of such implicit rightness. We can say that T'ai-Chi Ch'uan is a marvelous example of beauty and use and becomes a truthful experience when doing it.

Although the machinery of the human body is, needless to say, fantastically complicated and its structured action equally so, the coordinated resultant look in practicing is innocent, that is, harmonious, balanced, beautiful. The elasticity of the line of action, with its sensitive fluctuations of yin and yang and its intermeshing circlings, makes the body use itself, not only not superfluously but economically. Again we can take the working of a clock as an example and compare our structure to it, since rightness comes out of need, no matter how complicated the means.

The body is ultimately at its best when it is not felt. The painful back, the strained neck and shoulders make us know disagreeably the presence of those parts. Like a bridge which appears light and is so because the forces and stresses of its alignment are mathematically balanced, so the human being feels light and looks it when his muscles and joints behave correctly, in tune with each other. And when we are not conscious of the body, meaning the absence of irregularities, then the emotions are at their most neutral and, paradoxically, most pleasant, meaning the presence of harmony: well-being is, then, conscious, and vitality is at its maximum. Through its extraordinary discipline, T'ai-Chi Ch'uan helps each person to discover and create his own set of balances for the living of life.

In any work of art we expect to see a consistency as to its content, its substance, and its values. But even more than that, we expect to have a continuing gratification and pleasure from a work that is an art and from which we expect new profundities.

With T'ai-Chi Ch'uan, the more familiarity, the deeper its aspects, the richer its possibilities. To do it is to discover it anew, and to discover it is to penetrate its layers. No one submits himself to this exercise, as one does to a medicine: it is the spirit and the will power that must be willing. But then, according to my experience, T'ai-Chi Ch'uan is so artistically and emotionally persuasive that even the raw and ignorant beginner finds in himself a new will, a wish to do it, and pursue it.

In T'ai-Chi Ch'uan, the means is an end in itself. But also, like its philosophy, it is a beginning, a means for some other end, other purpose. It is a beginning in its application for a way in the conduct of life and work.

2. The Promise of Things to Come

When the player's experience is ripe enough to awaken certain qualities corresponding to the aims of T'ai-Chi Ch'uan—physical, mental, emotional—then the true meaning(s) of the Forms are explained and analyzed. It is at this time, when a high degree of maturity has arisen, that the nature of the symbolic names will have a "logical" reality as well as philosophical essence.

Despite the fact that the player may not be aware at first of any response higher than what results from the physical properties of the exercise, a kind of emotional and spiritual energy inevitably is being absorbed from the harmonious structure.

Although not consciously aware of "awareness," the active person-being, attentive to the requirements of the action, is involved with many simultaneous aspects of the exercise: the way the body moves; the flowing continuity of the movement; the "tempo" of the space-action; the relationship of balanced positions; the dynamic of yin-yang in energy and form; the coordinated combinations of patterns—all centers the mind and pleases the disposition. The structured part of the composition, at no matter what instant, becomes evident as being harmonious.

The technical method which the constant participation of the mind will disclose, bring forth, elements of feeling and perception not anticipated and certainly not prepared for. Such a development is inherent in the composite nature of T'ai-Chi Ch'uan.

It is quite evident that awareness of the various kinds of activity taking place is gradually increasing. Both mind attentiveness and physical proficiency produce newer experiences, sensed deeply. Such "knowingness" seemingly without boundary, does not, I hasten to say, arrive minute by minute, but surely and consistently appears—in due time—month by month.

At some point in this continuously progressing development, the student begins to become sensitive to the presence of the Forms as distinctive areas of attention, and naturally becomes inquisitive as to their meanings and significance in relation to the spirit of the whole.

The beginner had already been informed that the form names, as given, were symbolic of "other" kinds of qualities. The names, poetic or otherwise, were never to be thought of literally or done pantomimically; and were never to be taken at face value as images. The names were to be accepted as sign-posts, as guides, as references, in order to recognize certain defined positions (numbered as 108 Forms) "for the time being." Eventually, the metaphors, poetically symbolic, would be understood to be attributes, states of mind and feeling, all of which would be gradually attained since they were the aims and goals (the heart and soul) which would be naturally awakened in each player.

The true meanings encompassing mental, emotional, psychological, aesthetic-spiritual qualities eventually appear; through structured *action* (on all levels) and *not* through wishful, planned thinking; certain qualities grow, arise, and remain dynamically present.

Certain qualities are simple to discern when doing T'ai-Chi Ch'uan—such as becoming stronger, more certain of body coordinations, healthier—at the same time as becoming more patient and calm, but we can have no clue as to when we can attain them.

Results (full or partial) arrive at different times and vary for different people. All know that it is the *journey* through the activity in all its diversity, the *way* of the intricate harmony with space-time balance, form, and dynamic interplay that is the soil for the flowering of the exercise-aims.

The journey itself brings about, creates the well-being-ness in all the variety of its content, spiritual and physical.

Some of the qualities, developing step by step, are due to the player's mental application, diligence, and sensitive identification with the activity. They are (in brief):

Endurance, enhanced by physical strength
Flexibility and agility: quick reflexes
Perseverance—that is not self-conscious
Perceptivity—deepened
Ability to reject "negative emotions"
Greater awareness
Mental ease
Security in being attentive (and with oneself)
Greater insight and a higher degree of consciousness
And as written above—calmness, patience, centeredness.

These are promises to come—not from having been apprised of them by way of the symbolic meanings—but from the rich experience of doing and understanding the structure in its entirety. The player is being transformed, innocently; he or she becomes aware of these developing qualities by the *way* of the journey.

When the meanings of the Forms (each separately) are divulged or "unveiled" at the proper time, the player will recognize that those qualities have been felt and achieved—the quality of "self-being" and an expanding awareness—developed naturally and profoundly through the "universe" of T'ai-Chi Ch'uan. The player at this stage of mature well-being gradually perceives states of mind and feeling coming to life. This takes place constantly through the extraordinary structure of the exercise, which weaves a unity between the objective form (externally) and the subjective within.

The player can take it for granted that what will ultimately occur does not depend on certain explanatory words but on self-experience and knowledge of the way of the journey.

Does knowing the true meaning of each symbolic Form contribute anything to one's intelligent awakening? Absolutely, on yet another plane. More importantly, the player then appreciates the reason for *not* having been told, on the one hand, and on the other is being further enriched by the profundity, the richness of the metaphor—poetically symbolic, philosophically and artistically valid:—embedded in the symbol which stands not only for itself, but also for what it contains and does not reveal crudely and insensitively.

The player can then appreciate the Form as a wholeness terminating the previous transition and stirring the presence of another transition which moves into yet another culminating Form.

Comprehension of the various stages of growth advances one's consciousness and mental acumen—which (of course) leads to the Ultimate.

I shall now, without too much of a guilty conscience, reveal and analyze one Form to help the reader and the player understand the "insinuations" of a metaphor-symbol. I shall not, however, analyze or indicate its place in the evolutionary process of T'ai-Chi Ch'uan. (The Forms have many roles.)

"Grasping the Bird's Tail" is the second Form of the 108 and appears seven times (in the half-hour exercise). The Bird is the wren whose tail moves extremely quickly—so fast that it is almost impossible to touch or grasp it. (However, it *can* be done with the proper technique.) What is T'ai-Chi Ch'uan implying here? The perception is that all of us are trying to become more aware and through awareness "grasp" at consciousness, a most difficult procedure which takes times, effort, knowledge, technique, and understanding of the "problem." In other words, the name symbolizes the effort of trying to (grasp) attain a higher level of consciousness, which is as difficult as it would be to try to grasp the wren's tail. The metaphor extends the scope of imagination and of "nature" itself. The player throughout the entire exercise has been developing the state of awareness and hopes to find it easier to reach a higher level. The player does not need to know the meaning of the Form, because the ingredients of the whole composition "forces" the player to become aware, to a greater and greater degree, unwittingly, by means of its diversity and harmony.

Should the "new" player know its meaning beforehand, the process would be artificial and the connections made false. The overall effect is that one is gaining some awareness through, as has been mentioned, the entirety of the diverse activity which makes demands on one's attention—which in turn develops awareness and eventually lets us know that consciousness may be at hand—someday!

Every Form revealed as a unified whole deepens the perception of "Consciousness" and opens the way to a richer and more luminous experience of Body-Mind Harmony.

Acknowledgments

Several of the essays, comments, and poems here are reprints or revisions of writings published in *T'ai Chi Journal, Internal Arts Magazine, United Nations Secretariat News, Dance Observer, The Theatre Drama Review, Dance Scope, The Journal of Fredonia College, Dynamics Magazine, Dance Magazine, Show Business, United States-China People's Friendship Association Journal, Asian Music, Asian Arts, Ichpar,* and *Fighting Arts International.* The academic essay, "The Art of the Science of *T'ai Chi Ch'uan,*" appeared in *The Journal of Aesthetics and Art Criticism,* 25.4 (Summer 1967). Versions of several essays appeared in my *T'ai-Chi Ch'uan: Body and Mind in Harmony: The Integration of Meaning and Method.*

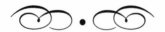

Also by Sophia Delza:
- *T'ai-Chi Ch'uan: Body and Mind in Harmony*
  (David McKay Publ: Denoel (Paris); paperback, Cornerstone Press (S&S))
- *Feel Fine, Look Lovely: The Dance-Art as Exercise*
  (Hawthorne Press)
- *T'ai-Chi Ch'uan: Integration of Meaning and Method*
  (State University of New York Press)
- Classic Chinese Theatre (in *Total Theatre* by E. T. Kirby
  E. P. Dutton & Co.)
- T'ai-Chi Ch'uan Record Album (Columbia Records of Columbia Pictures Corp.)

Illustration Credits

(in order of appearance)

Equanimity (Sophia Delza)

Alert Attention (People's Republic of China)

Attentive Stillness (Sophia Delza)

Opposites in Unity (courtesy of Rose Quong, author of Wit Wisdom and Written Characters [1944])

Timeless Ease (popular Scissors—Cut)

Structured Harmony (Photos—L. M. Lewicki)

Harmonious Diversity (Sophia Delza)

Peaceful Activity (newspaper clipping c. 1970s)

Ancient Formal Exercising Positions (People's Republic of China—New World Press)

Ancient Forms Active Today (People's Republic of China—New World Press)

T'ai-Chi Diagram (Ying Yang Balance, Body and Mind in Harmony)

Containment (Amsterdam Museum)

Index